LOVE FOR

ALWAYS *You*

'Knowing Chloe as a friend, I've always admired her strength, but seeing her pour her heart into *Always You* is beyond inspiring. She's turned her deepest challenges into a story of hope, love, and resilience that will touch everyone who reads it.'

– *Paris Hilton*

'This is the story of my dear friend Chloe who never stopped fighting for her dream of being a mum. Her journey through IVF heartbreak, love and sacrifice. It's a story full of strength, hope and the beautiful surprises life can bring.'

– *Elsa Pataky*

'Chloe's bravery in sharing her journey is truly inspiring. By speaking openly, she's helping to break down the silence around these experiences and giving strength to so many women. I'm in awe of her courage and honesty.'

– *Tash Oakley*

'A powerful, unflinching reminder that even in our darkest seasons, hope can bloom. Chloe's story is a lifeline for anyone navigating unseen battles – and proof that miracles are possible.'

– *Lisa Messenger*

'Chloe Fisher's *Always You* is a powerful story of loss, resilience, and the miracle of Bobbi. One that touched me deeply as someone who has walked a similar path, and a reminder of why stories like these matter so much.'

– Jesinta Franklin

'This is as real as it gets. No filters, no pretending. Chloe's journey has shown me that even when your heart is breaking and your world feels like it's falling apart, you can't give up!'

– Elyse Knowles

'This is Chloe – raw, brave, and unstoppable.'

– Paul Fisher

'I know this story like the back of my hand and still I was hanging off each word. Chloe's heart is on every page, a story of love, loss and longing.'

– Ellidy Pullin

'This book is more than a memoir – it's a gift of hope, love and strength. A moving reminder of the power of miracles.'

– Laura Enever

CHLOE FISHER

with ALLEY PASCOE

ALWAYS *You*

hachette
AUSTRALIA

Moonbeams and Rainbows used with the permission of Leanne Laydon.

hachette AUSTRALIA

Published in Australia and New Zealand in 2025
by Hachette Australia
(an imprint of Hachette Australia Pty Limited)
Gadigal Country, Level 17, 207 Kent Street, Sydney, NSW 2000
www.hachette.com.au

Hachette Australia acknowledges and pays our respects to the past and present Traditional Owners and Custodians of Country throughout Australia, and recognises the continuation of cultural, spiritual and educational practices of Aboriginal and Torres Strait Islander peoples. Our head office is located on the lands of the Gadigal people of the Eora Nation.

NATIONAL LIBRARY OF AUSTRALIA

A catalogue record for this book is available from the National Library of Australia

The authorised representative in the EEA is Hachette Ireland, 8 Castlecourt Centre, Dublin 15, D15 XTP3, Ireland (email: info@hbgi.ie)

ISBN: 978 0 7336 5392 6 (paperback)

Cover design and internal picture sections by Christabella Designs
Cover photograph by Karina Enever
Chloe Fisher author photograph by Karina Enever
Alley Pascoe author photograph by Alice Boshell
Typeset in 12.2/20 pt Scala Pro by Bookhouse, Sydney
Printed and bound in Great Britain by Clays Ltd, Elcograf S.p.A.

FSC www.fsc.org MIX Paper | Supporting responsible forestry FSC® C018072

Dedicated to Bobbi

CONTENTS

A NOTE FROM THE AUTHOR

There's a box I keep on a shelf, out of sight. Inside are three baby books. One is embossed with the word *Bump* on the front and *A Pregnancy Story* on the spine. Another is titled *Nine Months: The Beginning of You*.

The pages at the front of each book are lined with space to write down baby name ideas, advice from loved ones, parenting books and nursery plans. The middle is for weekly journal entries, tracing pregnancy cravings, waist measurements and doctor's appointments. On the last page, there's room for the baby's first photo, and all the details of their birth.

Inside the first book, which I bought in early 2020, I wrote, 'Positive test!!'

23/03/20

'Feeling normal, boobs are quite tender and big. Feeling a little tired but overall doing just fine!'

30/03/20

'Mum, Dad and Bump took our first road trip from Sydney to Currumbin. Started feeling a little bit of morning sickness, not pleasant. Spent some lovely time together down the beach. The ocean was so warm.'

15/04/20

'No heartbeat. Two ultrasounds and no baby in sight. Completely devastated.'

There are no more entries after that.

These books should be filled with happy memories, but I never got more than a few pages into them. They should be sweet keepsakes for my children, but instead, they're painful reminders. It hurts to look at the blank pages and think about what could have been.

I don't need these books to remember the pain of losing a pregnancy. I carry that pain with me every day. It's a pain so many women know all too well.

If you're reading this book, you might know this pain. You might be feeling it, drowning in it, or carrying it around with you, like I am.

People say motherhood is beautiful, but the road to it can be brutal. I know, because I've travelled that road for several years. For me, it was more like a steep obstacle course through the bush with dangerous valleys and hidden pits of quicksand. If you're currently on your own journey, I really want you to know you're not alone. Pregnancy loss and infertility can be isolating experiences. It's hard to talk about miscarriage, so we don't. Instead, we suffer in silence. We battle with shame. We feel alone.

At least, that's how I've felt at times. Logically, I know I'm not the only woman to lose a pregnancy. Studies show that up to one in five women who know they are pregnant will have a miscarriage. An estimated 110,000 women experience a miscarriage every year in Australia. I don't find any comfort in those numbers – it's devastating to know so many women are going through the same thing – but I have found comfort in other people's stories, in the arms of my friends, and in the community of women around me.

I hope you find some comfort in this book. As much as I want it to be a resource for hopeful parents, it's not a how-to guide. This is my personal story and lived experience of pregnancy, miscarriage and motherhood. In between chapters, I've included information, advice, mantras, reading material and practices that have helped me, in the hope they may help you too.

I am not a medical professional. I don't have a degree, and I certainly don't have all the answers. But I've spent years researching fertility, trying different treatments, speaking to doctors around the world, reading books and listening to experts. This is what I've learned, it's what I wish I had known from the beginning.

As you read my story and follow my fertility journey, the weight of the pain you're carrying may rest heavily on your shoulders. In those moments, please take care of yourself and go gently. If you need to put the book down and step away, do so. If you need to have a cry, call a friend or scream into a pillow, do so.

I've done all of the above: I've cried, called for help, screamed into the abyss. I've choked back tears reading pregnancy announcements on Instagram and then felt guilty for those tears. I've bitten my tongue when people have assured me 'It will happen when it's meant to happen,' or 'It just wasn't the right time,' or 'Have you tried relaxing?' There's no 'right' thing to say to someone experiencing infertility, but please don't say that. Telling a woman to relax has never, not once, made her relax.

I'm not going to tell you that everything happens for a reason. Those words are cold comfort in any traumatic moment.

This is what I will say, though:

I see you.

I hear you.

I am with you.

PROLOGUE

THE GRIEF BROUGHT ME TO MY KNEES. IT WASN'T THE FIRST time. And it wouldn't be the last. On an autumn day in 2022, I sank into the sand at Palm Beach on the Gold Coast. My husband, Paul, kneeled beside me, and we placed two long-stemmed, white roses into the footstep-imprinted sand in front of us. Two roses for two angels.

Two months earlier, I had been pregnant with two babies. I was no longer.

At the start of 2022, I wrote down my goals for the year. Number one on the list was: *Become a mother.* It was a goal I'd had for many years – my whole life, really. Paul and I had been actively trying for a baby for two-and-a-half years, and had experienced two miscarriages. So many twos. I desperately wanted 2022 to be the year I became a mother. I had such high hopes.

On Monday, 17 January, I started my fourth round of IVF injections. I injected myself twice a day, morning and night, every day for two weeks. Twenty days later, I had an egg retrieval procedure. Seven eggs were collected. Of those, five were inseminated, and two embryos survived until the all-important day-five mark. The last two embryos were given an A Grade, and I was told they were blastocyst, meaning they had developed and were hatching. My doctor told me they were some 'perfectly great looking embryos'.

'I've been doing this job for twenty-five years, and if this embryo doesn't work, I would be so surprised,' he said.

Medically, we were in a good position to conceive. Personally, I also felt like I was in a good place. It sounds a bit woo-woo, but I was trying hard to tune in to the universe and trust it. I asked for a sign. Specifically, I asked for a feather, as a symbol of hope.

That week, my mum, Alyson, was sitting on a bench under a tree outside her hairdresser, killing time before her appointment. She got talking to the couple sitting next to her – as Mum does – and opened up about what I was going through. Mum mentioned that we were looking for some positivity and a sign from above, before saying her goodbyes. You know, just a casual chat with strangers.

Fifteen minutes later, Mum was sitting in the hairdresser's chair when the couple walked in. 'We're just looking for the lady we met outside,' they told the receptionist, who pointed them in the right direction.

'Five minutes after you left, a feather dropped down and landed right where you were sitting. We thought you might want to know,' the couple explained.

A feather. A sign. A symbol of hope.

On the first day of February, I had a fresh Grade A embryo transferred into my uterus.

I took a pregnancy test earlier than I was meant to: eight days after my transfer. Two lines appeared. I was pregnant! I held onto those two lines for a couple of days before I worked up the courage to get my bloods taken to confirm the pregnancy and my hCG (human chorionic gonadotropin) levels. I was nervous; worried that the pregnancy test had been a false positive, that I wasn't really pregnant, that I had got my hopes up for nothing. When the blood test came back positive and my hCG levels confirmed it, I was so bloody excited. But still, the nerves remained.

There's a level of fear with every pregnancy, but after a loss, that fear is heightened. It is ever-present. No amount of excitement or joy or preparation can ease it. Trust me, I've tried.

Two weeks after having my pregnancy confirmed, I started intralipid treatment to help boost my immunity and fight off any bad cells that might want to attack the embryo. The procedure involved a fat emulsion being administered intravenously. It's often recommended for women with a history of early pregnancy loss and recurrent miscarriages.

I was doing everything humanly possible to give my pregnancy the best chance. As well as the intralipid, I was inserting progesterone (the pregnancy hormone), sometimes vaginally (if you know you know; not the most pleasant experience) and sometimes rectally, taking COQ10 and prenatal vitamins, doing acupuncture, meditating daily and crossing every bone in my body.

The bleeding started at 1 am. In the early hours of 26 February, I called Paul (who was working as a DJ overseas) in tears. My body went into shock, and I started shaking and vomiting. I never vomit, so that was a big deal. I secretly hoped it was morning sickness, but it felt different. My fear had become terror. *Not again, not again, not again,* I prayed.

When the sun rose, I booked in for an ultrasound with my fertility specialist, Dr Kee Ong. I cried the whole drive to the clinic. Inside, to my complete amazement, we saw a little heartbeat.

The bleeding eased, but the terror remained.

A scan the following week showed that the baby's heartbeat was still going strong. We also saw two sacs, which meant my pregnancy had been twins at one point, but only one baby remained alive. I didn't register the loss at the time – I was too focused on the little heartbeat inside me. I was still pregnant. That was all that mattered.

The rain started, and it didn't stop. At the end of February 2022, south-east Queensland was hit by one of the country's worst recorded flood disasters. The rain fell and the rivers rose. Roads went under, homes were lost, people were evacuated, supermarket shelves were emptied, and non-essential travel was restricted.

The region was devastated, and I was helpless. I was on bed rest, at Dr Ong's recommendation. I watched the news from bed in our house overlooking Palm Beach. Thankfully, Paul was back in Australia, and he and a group of his friends were out delivering essential items, rescuing people and animals in dinghies. As the days wore on, the death toll climbed; the loss was immeasurable. It was a heartbreaking time for everyone.

As the floodwaters began to recede, we were hit with more heartbreak.

On Wednesday, 9 March, Paul and I went into the clinic for our eight-week ultrasound. My bleeding had stopped and I was feeling pretty unwell, which I took as a good sign. Eight weeks was the furthest I'd got in a pregnancy. My first and second losses happened at around seven weeks. Because I'd made it further this time, I felt quite confident going into the scan.

That confidence faded as Dr Ong's face slowly dropped.

After a few minutes, he said, 'I'm sorry, I can't find a heartbeat.'

'No, no, no,' I said to Paul. 'Please no. Not again.'

Dr Ong sent me for a second ultrasound. I held onto a tiny bit of hope. *Maybe there was something wrong with Dr Ong's machine,* I thought. I prayed. I willed.

The waiting room at the second ultrasound appointment was full of visibly pregnant women. They were all admiring their sonogram pictures and subconsciously rubbing their bellies. It felt cruel. I desperately wanted to get out of that room, away from the bumps.

'It's so wrong,' I said to Paul, sitting in that room surrounded by everything we wanted, but couldn't have. I was crying and shaking when we were finally called into the ultrasound scan.

'I'm so sorry,' the nurse said. 'You should have been taken to a separate room. That shouldn't have happened.'

I tried to breathe through the sobs. When the screen beside me lit up, the scan showed our tiny twins right up close next to each other. Seeing the babies together was so special. It was the most beautiful image, but the sound didn't match.

There was no heartbeat.

They were both gone.

What the fuck?

Paul was devastated. I was confused. *Why does this keep happening?* I didn't understand.

Later that day, Dr Ong tried to give us some answers. We found out that the babies had been sharing a placenta, so the loss of the first one created a toxic environment for the second one. 'I know you're sick of being told you're just unlucky, but this was totally out of your control,' Dr Ong explained. 'It had nothing to do with your body, or your actions.'

On the drive home, every inch of my body ached. I don't know how my heart kept beating when it was so broken. I went home and wrote in my diary, 'We have now suffered three miscarriages and lost four babies. No words.'

The next day, I went in to have a D&C (dilation and curettage). I had booked in for the first available appointment and decided to go under anaesthesia for the procedure. Before they put me to sleep, someone told me they would send 'the product' off to be analysed. I felt sick. They weren't a 'product', they were my twins. My babies.

During the D&C, the doctor scraped the sides of my uterus and suctioned everything out. I simply couldn't bear the thought of having any remnants inside me. When I woke up from the anaesthesia, my uterus was empty.

I know I shouldn't have, but I felt like a failure. I felt like I had let Paul down. Again. I felt like the losses were my fault, like there was something wrong with me. Dr Ong had explicitly told me that wasn't the case, but I couldn't help feeling responsible. 'I'm so sorry, I'm so sorry,' I kept saying to Paul, who told me I had nothing to apologise for.

The whole thing hit Paul hard. He was meant to play two overseas shows that weekend, but he decided to cancel them to be with me. He wanted to post a personal message on Instagram apologising to his fans, and he told me he would say the cancellation was due to an urgent 'family matter'.

'Tell the truth,' I encouraged him. 'We need to talk about this. We need to acknowledge our babies.'

On 10 March, Paul shared that we had experienced another miscarriage. *I need to stay home to be there and support [my wife] right now while we go through this heartbreaking incident.*

The response was like nothing I've ever experienced. Both Paul and I were showered with love and support, from strangers and friends alike. I had more than 6000 people DM me. I was speechless. I still don't have the words to explain how grateful I am for all of those messages and the sheer kindness we were shown.

Three weeks later, I was still processing everything when Paul and I decided to go down to Palm Beach and pay tribute to our two angels with the two white roses. That day, we found out the babies had been identical twin boys. Before the loss, I had written a list of possible boy names in their baby book. Now, I didn't know if I would ever get to use one of those names. I didn't know how much more I could take.

That afternoon on the beach, our goddaughter, Minnie, sat on Paul's lap. She was five months old. Her mum, our friend Ellidy Pullin, didn't know if we would want to see Minnie after the miscarriage. She was worried it might be too painful. But seeing Minnie was all we wanted. She was a light in our lives when we so desperately needed it.

Ell had Minnie using sperm retrieved post-mortem from her long-time partner, Chumpy. Twenty months before we lost our baby boys, Ell lost the love of her life. He died in a shallow-water blackout while spearfishing in the water off Palm Beach, where we were remembering our identical twins. We remembered Chumpy, too.

'I know Chumpy is up there looking after your two boys, and your two other bubs,' Ell told me.

The grief brought us to our knees.

One

THE WAY WE WERE

THE IDEA CAME – AS THE BEST ONES OFTEN DO – OVER A FEW drinks with the girls. It was 2016 and I was with my closest friends on Sydney's Northern Beaches when we decided to make a time capsule. The plan was to open it in five years, but we forgot all about it. In early 2023, I was going through my filing cabinet (I know, I know, who owns a filing cabinet!?), and under 'F' for 'friendship', I found a handmade envelope. Inside were the notes we'd written seven years earlier and a photo of us from that time. We looked so young and innocent. We were.

There were six of us, including me and Ellidy. We wrote down silly things like our favourite song at the time (mine:

'Never Be Like You' by Flume featuring Kai, Ellidy's: 'Work' by Rihanna), and big things like our predictions for our futures.

For the question 'Where do you want to be in five years?' I wrote: 'Mum.'

It was all I had ever wanted in life. And my answer to that question, all those years ago, shows how long I've been dreaming about having a child.

On the notes we also listed, in order, who we thought would have kids first. We all wrote down my name first. It was a given. I was the 'mum' of the group, and we were all sure I would become a mum before anyone else. It wasn't something I'd ever questioned or doubted. I knew deep down in my bones I was going to be a mother. And so did my closest friends.

Growing up, I was the oldest of four kids. My parents, Alyson and David, had me in 1991, then my brother, Cooper, three years later. Olivia came along in 1996, and Sophia in 2000. I took my role as big sister very seriously. I'm a Leo, so naturally, I'm the organiser and leader of the siblings. I thought I was boss, and in a lot of ways I was. I kept my brother and sisters tightly under my wing when we were little.

My maternal instincts have always been strong. I don't know if I was born that way, or if I learned it from my own mum. I do know that my parents gave us the best childhood. We were so lucky. Dad is a draftsman and the most laid-back, easygoing, chill person I know. His motto is 'appreciation over expectation', and that's exactly how he lives. He's a creature of habit and follows the same routine every day: a cup of tea in bed, a stroll down to the beach to check out the surf, a ham-and-cheese toasted sandwich for lunch. Every. Day. Dad is a homebody, while Mum is a wanderer. She worked in film production before she had me, and became a stay-at-home mum after that, doing some cleaning jobs on the side. Mum loves to travel, whereas Dad prefers to stay in the same spot. They're opposites in that sense – she would like him to do more, and he would like her to do less – but they're made for each other. They really are soulmates. Don't get me wrong, they still piss each other off, but they love each other deeply. I grew up seeing – and feeling – that kind of love.

Together, Mum and Dad made a dynamite team. As parents, they were strict when they needed to be, but they also had a lot of trust and respect for us kids. They supported us unconditionally. We didn't have a lot of money, but we didn't struggle. It was a simple life. Our family holidays were spent road-tripping to Forster on the mid-coast of New South Wales, where we'd stay in a little holiday unit called South Sydney Juniors by the lake. Mum and Dad would load us kids into the Tarago, which didn't have air-con, and give us spray bottles of water to keep cool on the hot drive.

I lived in the same house in North Narrabeen all my life until I moved out of home. It was a six-bedroom house on a main road with a long set of steps down to the front door. I have happy memories of playing with my neighbours, who were the same age as me and Cooper. We used to make up 'clubs', like the gardening club, where we would go to houses on our street and weed their gardens for pocket money. Then there was the backyard book club, where I charged a 50-cent membership fee. I was always the leader of these groups.

My mum's parents and her nan (my grandparents and great-grandmother) lived a couple of suburbs over and I spent a lot of time with them. I was the first grandchild, so I felt lucky to have one-on-one time with them. Grandma and Poppa took me to Disneyland in California when I was two-and-a-half. Cooper was a baby, so he stayed at home with Mum and Dad while I had my grandparents' undivided attention. They spoiled me the way grandparents do, and were very involved in my childhood.

I was always small for my age. When I started school – at Narrabeen North Public School, which was at the end of my street – I was the littlest one there. I met my best friend, Laura Enever, on the first day of kindergarten. She was a sporty blonde tomboy, and I was a girly brunette. We were so bloody cute. From the moment we met, we did everything together: gymnastics, acrobatics, tumbling and surfing. Laura was always the best at whatever we did; I never came close.

I wasn't super athletic, but I danced and played netball (on the wing; I was too short for defence). I did try my hand at being a little surfer grommet like Laura – and also Cooper – but an incident involving seaweed put an end to that. We were at a girls' Boardriders Club event when I got smashed by a wave and held under the water. When I finally came up for air, I was all tangled up in seaweed. Spooked, I decided surfing wasn't for me.

I was more academic than sporty. I loved English and Maths, and I cared a lot about doing well at school. I worked hard in class, always submitted my homework on time and followed the rules. I was such a perfectionist, and I used to stress out over exams and assignments. I hated to be in trouble, so I never rebelled. I was probably a bit of a goody-two-shoes if I'm honest. I certainly looked the part, with ribbons in my hair, and my neat, tidy uniform.

My favourite photo of me as a kid is one of me and Laura, dressed up as the Spice Girls. Our mums were good friends, and they had decided to send us to audition for the talent segment on the TV show *Hey Hey It's Saturday*. We choreographed a dance routine and got all done up in pop star outfits. I was Sporty Spice (purely because I had brown hair) and Laura was Baby Spice (again, for hair colour reasons). We didn't make it onto the show – our mums still insist it must have been rigged – but it was worth it for the photo.

Laura is my oldest and closest friend, my ride or die. She is the most caring, empathetic and generous person ever. If more people were like Laura Enever, the world would be a better place. I know my world is better with her in it. As well as having each other, we also had a great group of mates around us. We all used to walk to school together: me, Laura, Maia, Elly, Bridget, Kate and Maddy.

Despite having such good friends, I wasn't a big fan of sleepovers as a kid. Much like my dad, I'm a homebody and I love routine. Whenever I tried to stay over at a friend's house, I'd get anxious and ask to be picked up. This was back before mobiles were a thing, so I'd have to get my friend's mum to call my mum so I could go home. Every. Single. Time.

I didn't remember this when I first sat down to write this book. It wasn't until I started reflecting on my childhood and talking to my mum about it that she reminded me of my panic attacks. I went through a bout of anxiety at the end of primary school and the start of high school. It got so bad that Mum took me to the hospital when I was having a panic attack and hyperventilating. They gave me a paper bag to breathe into. The doctors couldn't find anything physically wrong with me, so they sent me home.

Even now, I don't know what I was so anxious about. As I've said, I had a happy childhood with the best parents and the greatest friends. I didn't have a reason to be anxious, but I was. I've tried to make sense of it. I know there is a history of mental illness in my family. I know I was a real mummy's girl, and probably struggled with separation from her. And I know I put a lot of pressure on myself to do well at school.

The thing with anxiety is that it doesn't need a reason. It doesn't discriminate. Even the most externally put-together people can suffer internally.

Just as I don't know why I was consumed with anxiety, I don't know how I climbed my way out of it, either. I'm thankful that my anxiety didn't get worse, or evolve into depression. Instead, it lifted. Like a feather in the wind.

I was never going to be a supermodel. My height wouldn't allow it. But that didn't stop my mum from entering me in kids' modelling competitions when I was young. I did catwalks and catalogues. I was a child model for Best and Less, and the hand and foot model for Avon. I do have really nice hands and feet.

After years of doing shoots and shows, I wanted to take my modelling further. I met with one of the big agencies in Sydney and their feedback was brutal: 'You're too little, but also too big,' they told me. I was too short and weighed too much to model. What a double whammy.

I'm glad I had a healthy body image and decent self-esteem. Those comments could have knocked the confidence out of me – and I'm sure they did for a moment – but I was comfortable in my own skin. I've always cared about my appearance, but I'm not consumed by it. Feeling fit and healthy is more important to me than being skinny or perfectly in proportion.

I didn't grow up knowing what I wanted to be. After ruling out modelling, I figured I would become a school teacher. I think lots of kids consider teaching because it's the industry they're most exposed to. I didn't have a deep desire to be an educator, but I loved kids and thought teaching would be achievable. In saying that, I didn't really want to go to university. Getting a degree to frame and hang on my wall wasn't something I dreamed about. Still, I cared about school and wanted to graduate with a good mark.

I started high school at Narrabeen Sports High, which, again, was super close to my home. As the name suggests, it was a school of athletes. Rugby, AFL, soccer and surfing could all be taken as subjects. Naturally, Laura excelled. I didn't. I never felt like I fit in at Narrabeen Sports High. I took the academic subjects seriously, but it felt like no-one else did. The other kids only cared about sports, and would piss about in class. That wasn't me.

I was in PE one day in Grade Eight when a boy in my class pulled my pants down. I was horrified. I never went back.

In Grade Nine, I started at Mater Maria Catholic College in Warriewood. I had friends who went there, which made it easier to start at a new school. The cute uniform helped, too. At Mater Maria, I was in the same grade as Ellidy, but we didn't hang out in the same friendship group. Ell hates it when I say this, because we're so close now, but we weren't close friends back then. If anything, we were acquaintances. We knew each other and had mates in common, so we crossed paths – as did everyone on the Northern Beaches.

There's a reason they call the Northern Beaches of Sydney the insular peninsula. It's like a big, small town. Everyone knows everyone. The ocean brings people together. Even though I gave up on surfing after the seaweed incident, I still spent most weekends at the beach.

When we were around fourteen, Laura and I were both sponsored by the surfwear brand Roxy. She surfed for them, and I modelled for them. Sometimes we'd model together. Those campaigns were my favourite. It's pretty special to have professional photos of us at that age to look back on.

The older I get, the more reflective I am. When I try to remember my 2016 self – the girl building a time capsule over drinks with her mates – it's hard to recognise her. I'm a completely different person now; I've evolved in ways I'd never imagined. But the one thing that's remained the same is my desire to be a mum.

A guide to your very own time capsule

On your own or with a group of friends, answer the following questions openly and honestly on a piece of paper. Then hide the note somewhere safe and forget all about it. Set a reminder for five years' time to find the piece of paper and reflect on how life has changed, what you've learned and how far you've come.

Write down:

- Today's date
- Current outfit of choice
- Song that's on repeat
- Your current line of work
- What you hope to do for work in five years
- Three goals
- Your three favourite things to do daily
- Something you want to say to your future self
- The last big headline that really caught your attention

Two

MAGNETS

It was totally out of character. I don't know what came over me. Actually, that's not true. I know exactly what came over me: three $1 'Double Double' shots – a lethal mix of vodka, Red Bull and an Extra Joss caffeine sachet. I was in Bali on a girls' trip in 2012, and we were running amok at Alleycats Bar just off Poppies Lane in Kuta. Standing at the bar, I made eye contact with the hot surfer across the room.

It wasn't the first time I'd seen him. The day before, Paul Fisher rode past me and my friends on his scooter outside our hotel in Legian. I checked him out because he was a spunk; one of my friends did a double-take because he recognised him as an Aussie surfer on the qualifying tour. 'Oi, that's that Fisher guy,' my friend noted.

I had heard of the infamous Fisher because my brother and several of my friends were also on the qualifying tour. He had a reputation as a cheeky larrikin, and he was making a name for himself in certain circles. But it wasn't his reputation or his name that drew me to him. It was his blond surfy hair and dreamy blue eyes.

When I saw those eyes across the bar at Alleycats, I couldn't help myself. I gave Paul a nod and a wink. That's all it took. We were on.

I sidled up to him and started a conversation. 'So, what are you up to tonight?'

'Just a quiet one. I'm having some meatballs and heading home,' Paul said.

'Like fuck you are. You're not going anywhere,' I replied, ordering another round of Double Doubles.

Paul later told me he was happily taken aback. He wasn't used to having a girl chat him up – usually, it was the other way around. I'd turned the tables on him, and he was rather pleased by the flipped script.

Within twenty minutes, I was sitting on Paul's lap. Photos from that night show us being tourists and posing on the Kuta surfboard, and later, dancing up a storm in the cages at the iconic Bounty Club. So much for Paul's quiet night! Looking at those pictures, you'd think we'd been together forever, not that we'd only just met. There was an easiness between us straight away. It wasn't something I'd ever felt before, and it wasn't something I had been seeking out.

I had recently come out of a long-term relationship. I met Jack when I first started going to Mater Maria Catholic College. He was in the same grade as me and we coupled up. After school, we moved in together in an apartment in Mona Vale. We were going through the motions: finish school, move out, grow up. We'd been together five or six years when we both decided we wanted to see what else was out in the world. We didn't know a life outside of our relationship, and we were curious to explore the possibility. We mutually ended things and are still friends today.

Naturally, the first thing I did as a newly single twenty-year-old was book a girls' trip to Bali.

The night I met Paul, I went back to his hotel. He was sharing with a group of guys from Maroubra, who I knew from my days hanging out there with my mum's sister, Kylie. I am not being a princess when I say that Paul's accommodation was feral. It was actually disgusting. There were cockroaches in the cupboards, green slime in the pool and a damp smell that nearly made me gag. Still, I stayed there for a few days with Paul and the boys. The things you do for love, eh? It was a full-blown holiday romance. But after a few days in a love bubble in the hotel from hell, I started to wonder what on Earth I was doing. I was on a girls' trip! I shouldn't be shacked up with a guy!

I went back to my friends in Legian, and we got on with the rest of our holiday. Somehow, Paul kept showing up wherever I was. We didn't plan it. We would magically end up at the same cafe or bar and find ourselves naturally relaxing into each other. We were like magnets, pulling together whenever we got close.

It's not like we were checking each other's Instagram stories – this was before smartphones and social media. Paul had a Blackberry, for god's sake (that makes me feel ancient).

Anyway, I ruined Paul's quiet night, and he ruined my girls' trip. We spent three weeks orbiting each other in Bali, and in that time, it felt like I got to know the real Paul. Not 'Fisher', but Paul – the man behind the moniker. Even though Paul is known for being a character and the centre of attention, he's actually a really private person. He was born in Bundaberg, Queensland, but when he was little, he moved to South Africa, where his mum worked in the casino industry. Paul's parents split when he was a baby. His dad had more to do with his older brother, whereas Paul's mum raised him on her own. She worked her arse off to provide for her boys, and she did such an amazing job raising them.

When Paul was ten, they moved back to Queensland and settled at Broadbeach on the Gold Coast. His older brother went to boarding school, so it was just Paul and his mum at home. He says he had an epic childhood, riding his bike around town, surfing and hanging out with heaps of mates.

He describes himself as a little Dennis the Menace, always conveniently rocking up whenever someone was having a barbecue. The more I learned about Paul, the more I wanted to know.

There was an undeniable connection between us. But as our time in Bali came to an end, I figured our romance would too. Paul was living in California then, busy competing on the qualifying series, and my life was in Sydney. I was working in advertising in the city and absolutely loving it. He was a broke surfer, and I was in a relatively new job with no annual leave left. We weren't likely to see each other again in person anytime soon.

The conversation went something like this: 'Look, this has been so lovely. I literally love spending time with you, but you live in America, and I live in Australia, so I can't see how it's going to work.'

We said goodbye without knowing when – or if – we'd see each other again. I wondered 'if'. Paul knew it was only a matter of 'when'. He was sitting on the plane on the tarmac waiting for his flight to take off when he messaged one of my friends. *Tell that chick I'm in love with her,* he said.

She's into you too, my friend replied.

Paul smiled the whole flight back. His face was sore by the time he landed.

Despite being on opposite sides of the world and in different time zones, we spoke every day. I told my brother about the bloke I met in Bali who I was still talking to. 'His name is Paul Fisher,' I said.

'It better not be the Paul Fisher I know,' Cooper replied, picturing the good-time surfer he knew from the scene. 'Hard no. He's not the kind of guy for you, Chlo.'

I insisted Paul was really sweet and cool, but Cooper, having three sisters, wasn't having a bar of it. He was in over-protective brother mode.

In the States, Paul was having conversations about me too. Laura was over there for a surf comp, and he sought her out. 'I'm going to marry your friend Chloe one day,' he told her.

She rolled her eyes. 'You wish.'

'Mark my words,' he said. 'That's the woman I'm going to marry.'

We'd been talking every day for several months when Paul told me he was going pig hunting with some friends on a remote island in Hawaii, so he'd be out of reception for a few days. I didn't think anything of it. I had no idea he'd secretly reached out to my brother to get my home address (under the guise of sending me flowers), or that he'd booked a flight from Hawaii to Sydney. Because the universe is so small, Cooper's then-girlfriend Erika was on the same flight as Paul, and they recognised each other. 'You cannot tell anyone I'm on this flight,' Paul said to Erika, before asking how she was getting from the airport to the Northern Beaches.

Erika's dad was picking her up, so Paul bummed a lift with them.

When Erika's dad pulled up in the pick-up zone, Paul loaded an XXL surfboard bag onto the roof of the car – a convertible SAAB. The roof sank under the weight.

'Who is this guy?' Erika's dad said with his eyebrows raised.

Erika shrugged. 'I really don't know. Can we just drop him at the Chapmans' house?'

I wasn't home when Paul made it to Narrabeen. I remember Mum messaging me asking when I was coming home. 'I'm not,' I replied. 'I'm going to Laura's after work and we're going out to dinner.'

Little did I know, Paul had showed up on my doorstep with his suitcase and his board bag. When Mum answered the door, totally confused, Paul tried to explain. 'Um, hi. I'm here to see Chloe.'

'She's not here,' Mum said, looking Paul up and down questioningly. Still, Mum dutifully drove the stranger on her doorstep down to Laura's once she knew that's where I was heading. I hadn't even planned on going in, I was just going to pick Laura up on the way to dinner, but when I pulled up out the front and messaged her, she insisted I come inside. 'I've got something to show you,' she said.

Ugh. Fine. I dragged myself into Laura's place, annoyed at the effort. I let myself in and walked over to Laura, who was sitting at the dining table. 'Are you nearly ready?' I rushed her.

She started to answer me when I turned around and saw Paul standing there. I couldn't believe it. My Bali heartthrob was standing right in front of me, in Sydney, in my best friend's dining room.

I started running on the spot in disbelief. I jumped into his arms and squealed with excitement. I never wanted our hug to end. We held each other so tight; I think part of me was checking to make sure he was real and not a figment of my imagination. When we finally came up for air, Paul sat down next to Laura at the table and pulled me onto his lap. It was just like our first night together at Alleycats; me sitting on his lap, him wrapping his arms around my waist. We've been together ever since.

I packed my life into a suitcase, said goodbye to my friends and family and headed to the States. After Paul surprised me in Sydney, we spent a few weeks together, living in the front room of my parents' house – I know, how romantic – and celebrated our first Christmas with each other. We both knew we were going to be together. When Paul left to go back to America in March 2013, I followed him. I didn't know how long I would stay overseas, but I knew I wanted to give our relationship a red-hot chance.

It was a huge move for me. I had lived in the same pocket of the Northern Beaches my entire life. It was hard for me to leave my job, too, but I wasn't going to just sit around in Narrabeen, waiting for Paul to come home. I was going to make a go of things in the States.

I've always been a worker. Remember the gardening club and backyard book club I started for pocket money? I got a 'real' job as soon as I could. It was the dream gig for a thirteen-year-old – working behind the counter at the local Baker's Delight. I was so little, the apron dead-set touched the floor and wrapped around my waist three times. I used to come home with bags of bread rolls and finger buns and take them to school the next day to give to the boys in my grade. No wonder I had a lot of friends.

After Baker's Delight, I worked at a juice shop and then at Woolworths, and I babysat and nannied on the side as well. When I finished school, I still didn't really know what I wanted to do, so I applied to be a flight attendant. As you do. I got accepted by Jetstar and went to Melbourne for a month for ground school. There was so much to learn. Each flight attendant position has different rules and responsibilities, but everyone needs to know every inch of the plane, every storage compartment and every safety protocol. I was in my element, studying all the manuals and learning everything there is to know.

When I passed ground school, I was offered a domestic role with Jetstar. I mostly flew between Sydney and the Gold Coast. Back and forth, back and forth. I figured I would climb the ranks and eventually end up flying internationally. I loved that every day – and every flight – was different. Of course, the very best thing was getting to wear the uniform.

I had been flying for less than a year when I hurt my shoulder on the job and had to give it up. It sucked, but I wasn't devastated – I'd never had a burning passion to be a flight attendant. It was my job, not my dream.

On the ground, I reached out to a friend of my mum's who worked at ACP Magazines and scored a job in the advertising department. The offices were on Park Street in the city, so I'd get dressed up and do my make-up, then catch the 7 am bus from North Narrabeen into the CBD. I thought I'd made it, prancing through the city in my heels, going to important meetings and travelling the country to meet with clients. It was epic.

I was still working at ACP in 2012 when I went to Bali on that fateful girls' trip. After meeting Paul and deciding to give things a go in the States, I left my job. I was never going to be a kept girlfriend, though – I was too independent. Also, Paul lost his surfing sponsorship not long after we got together.

It was a turning point for both of us. We were both standing at a fork in the road, but we weren't carving a new path on our own. We had each other. Paul decided to move on from surfing and pursue his passion for music. He'd been DJing surf parties for years, and he wanted to give the profession a serious go.

I saw Paul back himself and decided to do the same. I was going to launch something of my own. I borrowed $5000 from Paul – the last of his savings – and $5000 from my grandparents, who knew I would pay them back straight away, and used the money to start a swimwear brand. I didn't know a thing about business, but I knew a lot about bikinis. After all, I'd spent the majority of my life in swimmers. Once I had the idea – fully reversible, seamless and skimpy-cut swimwear – I made it happen. I launched Aloé Swimwear – pronounced al-oh-ee – in mid-2013 from my new base in the States. The business name was made up of the first initials of my mum Alyson's name, and the last two of mine. Mum and my sisters handled logistics in Australia while I was overseas.

Paul and I moved into a rental in Oceanside in Northern California, near San Diego. He had his first professional (non-surf event) gig in the city. I was there, front and centre, cheering him on. It was . . . an experience. The venue didn't have a liquor licence, so they weren't actually allowed to have a live music act. To get around this, they put Paul behind an LED screen. He couldn't see the dance floor or feel the energy of the crowd. Instead, I reported back to him. *It's so fucking good babe,* I messaged him.

It was the first of many gigs, and the start of my official role as a hype girl.

I was trying to make the most of being in America. Ellidy turned twenty-one in May, so we did a big girls' trip to Mexico, hitting Tulum and Cancun, before winding up in Las Vegas. Ell was seeing a guy named Chumpy. Well, his name was Alex Pullin, but everyone called him Chumpy. They'd officially met at Laura's twenty-first, six months earlier. He was a professional snowboarder and spent a lot of time travelling on the snow circuit, so I'd only met him a couple of times. But I didn't need to know Chumpy well to know Ell was smitten. I remember being in a Vegas hotel room when Chumpy's birthday present for her arrived. It was a song he'd written for her.

There was a line in the song that went, 'I've got the strongest feeling, my love has found its home in your heart.' How bloody beautiful is that? We all jumped around the room, dancing and squealing along to Ellidy's birthday song from her lover.

Meanwhile, back in California, my surfy boy was making music too. When all the girls went back to Australia, I went home to Paul in Oceanside. We shared our rental there with Paul's childhood mate and fellow surfer Leigh 'Sedz' Sedley and his girlfriend Alicya. Paul and Sedz formed the DJ duo Cut Snake (as in, mad as a cut snake – get it?). The boys were giving music their all. I was splitting my time between launching Aloé and travelling back and forth across Los Angeles for Cut Snake gigs with the boys and Alicya.

The boys weren't making a lot from their shows, and whatever they did earn had to be split between the two of them and cover management fees and travel costs, so we were barely getting by. I know everyone says they come from humble beginnings, but these were really humble beginnings.

The four of us would trek to a far-flung corner of Cali and stay in the cheapest motel we could find near the venue. These places were usually rank, and sometimes a bit dodgy. We roughed it, but we drew the line at some things. Some nights Sedz and Alicya stayed in their camper in a car park to save money on a motel room, but Paul and I chose to have a double bed and a shower. Oh, the luxury.

Still, I loved watching Paul play. I find it incredible how he gets excited for every single show, even if there are only five people in the crowd, and I'm one of them. His energy when he's behind the decks is like nothing else. It's pure passion.

DJs get a lot of shit for 'just pushing buttons', but I've seen firsthand the amount of work and commitment that goes into it. It doesn't matter if Paul is sick or exhausted, he plays rain, hail or shine. He gives the same level of love to that crowd of five as he does to a thumping festival mosh pit. He *always* puts on a performance. I admire him for that.

Paul's gigs took us to Hawaii, to a cruise ship off Miami, and back to Bali, where it all began. My swimwear label took us to Bali too, because that's where all my pieces were manufactured. We didn't have much, except for each other and our passports, but we did the best we could with what we had.

As much as I loved seeing Paul giving his DJ dreams a go, I struggled a lot in those early days. I'm such a homebody – I like the comfort of my own bed – so being on the road for shows was hard for me. I was also homesick for Sydney and my family. I felt like I'd given up my whole world to join Paul in America, and that made our relationship feel uneven. Nothing felt secure to me, and I hated being in limbo.

The DJ life was fun, but I knew I wanted to settle down sooner rather than later. I wanted a husband and a family, and I thought that meant having a white picket fence. I craved stability, but chaos continued to find me.

I told Paul early on that I wanted to have kids. I was only twenty-one, but I wasn't opposed to being a young mum. When we spoke about starting a family, Paul said, 'Let's live a little first.' He wanted to do more travelling and get ahead in his career before bringing a child into the world. I understood. I was sure it would happen when it was meant to happen.

Three

DREAMS

It was a stinking hot Saturday afternoon in the Colorado Desert, April 2018. Paul was playing Coachella for the first time, and he was about to debut a new song. Under the DoLab Tent, he turned to us – me; Brett, his manager; Cody, his agent and James, his publicist – standing behind him on the tiny stage. 'Watch this.' Paul said. Then he played his recently completed track, 'Losing It', to the sweaty crowd. The crowd went wild. He brought them to the edge and then pushed them over it. It was the exact reaction Paul was hoping for, and our friend Angelo caught it all on camera.

'I've not seen that reaction from a first ever play of a record in a long time,' James said later. The video of the performance went crazy online, and the song went on to become the biggest dance track of the summer, and then of the decade.

Everyone at Coachella was talking about it. When another artist pulled out of playing the Yuma Tent the next weekend of the festival, Paul got the call-up. Word had spread among the festivalgoers about 'this Fisher fella', and his tent packed out. It was at capacity, people literally started crawling under the tent to see Paul play. It was wild. I was so proud.

Coachella was one of Paul's first solo shows as Fisher. After a few years playing as Cut Snake, Paul decided to go out on his own, under the moniker of his last name. His debut single was aptly titled 'Ya Kidding' (a phrase he uses all the time), and his first EP was called 'Oi Oi'. When Paul struck out on his own, we moved out of the Oceanside place we'd been sharing with Sedz and Alicya and got a tiny apartment under the Hollywood sign, just the two of us. The crowd's reaction at Coachella was a sign that Paul was onto something.

Still, Paul didn't let the moment go to his head. Just after Coachella, we headed to China for his debut playing at Electric Daisy Carnival (EDC). Paul played a side stage and put on a hell of a show with all the theatrics: fog, flames and pyrotechnics. He used his full bag of tricks, to a crowd of . . . two people. I kid you not, there were only two people in the audience. We tried to keep the memory of Coachella front of mind.

While Paul was finding his place and rhythm in music, I was gaining traction in business. Aloé Swimwear went global within nine months of launching – Ellidy was my first ever customer – and we picked up the huge retail chain General Pants as an Australian stockist. When we launched the second collection, our exclusive one-piece sold out (bar three pieces) in the first three hours.

It felt like both Paul and I were gaining momentum in our careers. More importantly, we were going strong as a couple, too. From the moment we met, we've been two peas in a pod. We just really like being around each other. If I'm running errands, he'll come with me because we're happiest when we're together. We're a solid unit. We never want to be apart.

Don't get me wrong, we still fight and bicker. I'm a self-confessed neat freak, but Paul is next level. He is obsessive. He will vacuum and clean every single day. He can't not. If there's a used bowl in the sink, he'll need to wash it up – he won't be able to think of anything else until that bowl is clean and put away. His need for tidiness is all-consuming, and it can cause issues between us. I like a pristine house as much as the next girl, but not at the cost of sanity.

The biggest issue between us, though, was our location. After four years living out of a suitcase, I missed home more than ever. Every time Paul and I came back to Narrabeen and stayed at my parents' house with all my siblings, the pull got stronger. I told Paul how much I wanted to go back and live on the Northern Beaches again. He had no connection to the area, so he wasn't as keen, but we found a compromise.

We started renting a studio apartment out the back of a friend's place on Narrabeen Lake as our Australian base. I say studio apartment, but it was really a shack. The joint was ridiculously small. I kid you not, the lounge was so close to the oven, you could flip your eggs sitting on the couch. It was me, Paul and my childhood dog Lola living in this teeny tiny apartment. I wouldn't have wanted to be anywhere else, or with anyone else.

Narrabeen was home. It was where my mum, dad, siblings and most of my mates were. No matter how far away I travelled, I was always drawn back to Narrabeen. Paul felt the same way about the Gold Coast. 'I want to raise my kids on the Goldy,' he told me, more than once.

It was exciting to picture little mini-Fishers growing up on the beaches on the Gold Coast.

Change was on the horizon, I could feel it.

In July 2018, Paul released 'Losing It' as an official single. It went on to hit Number One on Billboard's Dance Club Songs chart, was nominated for a Grammy and took out second place in the Triple J Hottest 100.

That song changed everything for us.

I was sunbaking on the deck of a superyacht on Pittwater. Yes, I know how bourgeois that sounds, and it absolutely was. It was the start of 2019, and Paul and I were back in Australia.

Friends from America had come over to spend New Year's Eve watching the fireworks on the aforementioned superyacht on Sydney Harbour. Paul had a NYE show in Melbourne, and normally I would have been there, but I chose the superyacht over him. Sorry, babe!

Paul joined us on 1 January, and we celebrated the beginning of a new year together. Little did I know, we were about to have another reason to celebrate.

Over the next couple of days, we sailed the yacht from Sydney Harbour to Pittwater on the Northern Beaches. That's where we were pulled up, in a secluded bay, when I was sunbaking. I noticed one of our mates had started filming me, and then I saw Paul come up the stairs to the top deck. I was sure I was about to be pranked. 'What are you gonna do?' I asked him with a grin.

Instead of stitching me up, he opened a ring box.

'What do ya reckon?' Paul said, nodding to the most beautiful diamond ring I've ever seen.

My hands went straight to my mouth. I couldn't believe it. I crawled over to Paul and kissed him. 'Holy shit, are you kidding?' I said as he put the ring on my finger. 'I'm engaged!'

Paul had planned a whole speech and wanted to get down on one knee, but his nerves got the better of him. 'What do ya reckon?' is all he could manage. He had been carrying that ring box around since before Christmas, when he was originally planning to propose in front of my family. Paul 'did the right thing' and asked my dad for his blessing; he knew not to ask my mum because she can't keep a secret to save her life.

They were walking down Narrabeen Beach to go for a surf when Paul worked up the courage to tell Dad he wanted to propose. 'I've got something to ask you,' Paul said nervously. 'I love your daughter, and I love you guys, and I hope you don't mind if I ask her to marry me.'

Dad shook Paul's hand, then gave him a hug. It makes my heart happy to think about that moment; my two favourite men embracing on the beach. Paul had the green light, but he decided not to propose on Christmas Day because he wanted our engagement to be its own celebration. Instead, he carried the ring box around for more than a week, waiting for the right moment.

By 3 January, he couldn't wait any longer. 'Fuck it, I'm going to propose to Chloe right now,' he told our friend on the yacht, bringing him in to film the moment.

It was the best day of my life. I was desperate to tell everyone the happy news, but we had no phone reception in the middle of the bay, which meant we got to just enjoy the moment together.

That night, the boat pulled into Palm Beach, where we had dinner at Dunes. My family and close friends, including Laura, were there waiting for us with champagne. I had never been happier. Being engaged felt so surreal, but also so right. I had a sense that this was just the beginning; like we were starting the rest of our lives together. We were going to get married and have a family, just like I had always dreamed.

Life was good. At the beginning of 2019, we split our time between Narrabeen, the Gold Coast, where Ellidy and Chumpy had just bought a place and were settling in, and Margaret River in Western Australia, where our friends were getting married.

We planned our WA trip down to the minute. The wedding happened just before the Grammys, which were held in LA (a *long* way from WA) and we couldn't miss either event. 'Losing It' was up for Best Dance Recording. We were going to the Grammys, even if we had to hire a small plane to fly us from the wedding to Perth so we'd arrive in time. And that's exactly what we did. We organised a charter plane from a small airstrip near the wedding venue to take us to Perth airport, where we would board our flight. The airstrip was so small, we had to board the plane before sunset because it couldn't take off in the dark. We made it with minutes to spare.

'Where's my backpack?' Paul asked me.

'Fuck.'

It was a summer's day, and I'd taken Paul's backpack out of the car and put it inside our accommodation because I didn't want his laptop to overheat. The backpack had our passports in it. We couldn't leave without it.

Paul raced back to the house and the pilot agreed to make a pitstop at a bigger airstrip further away so we could pick

Paul up en route once he had our passports. I boarded the tiny plane, and Paul drove up and down the runway beeping the horn and flashing his lights to scare away the kangaroos on the airstrip so we could take off.

Job done, Paul fanged it as fast as he could. In the air, all I could do was pray that he was fast enough.

He was, in fact, too fast. The cops pulled him up on the highway on the way to the second airstrip. The timing could not have been worse. Before the police officer could even ask Paul why he'd been driving so fast, he pleaded his case.

'I'm so fucking sorry to do this. I know it's rude and wanky, but you really need to let me go right now because I'm late for a flight to the Grammys,' he explained. 'I'm nominated for a Grammy. I can't miss the Grammys. It's the Grammys!'

For whatever reason – confusion, pity or Aussie pride for a local act – the cop waved Paul on. He made it. We landed in LA three hours before we were due on the red carpet. I rushed through hair and make-up and arrived at the Staples Center in a whirlwind. Only then did I breathe out – for the first time since I'd left Margaret River.

I was the world's proudest fiancée watching Paul do interviews on the red carpet. When *Sunrise* TV reporter Edwina Bartholomew stopped Paul for a chat, she warned him not to swear on the live cross back to Australia. 'You're a superstar in the dance world,' she said to him.

'Oh, I don't know about that. Not yet,' Paul replied modestly. 'I'm just pushing the buttons and going fucking . . . Oops!'

Oops, indeed. Someone posted a video of the interview online. It got over a million views.

'Losing It' didn't end up winning the Grammy – I swear Paul was robbed! He deserved to win. But it didn't make me any less proud of him. We celebrated hard, regardless.

Paul hosted a Grammys afterparty with Diplo at a mansion in the Hollywood Hills. It was like something out of a movie, seriously. Leonardo DiCaprio and Katy Perry were there. Ya kidding!

There were more pinch-me moments to come throughout the year. There was Carnival in Rio de Janeiro, Coachella in Cali, EDC in Vegas, and Paul's first time playing Ibiza in Spain. Somehow, amid all that travel and adventure, we found time to plan a wedding.

We knew we wanted our big day to be in Bali, where we first met and fell in love. And we knew we wanted it to be one hell of a party. We invited all our closest people and not a single person declined. Everyone wanted to be a part of the celebrations – all 172 guests.

We were lucky to know the owner of The Lawn, a stunning restaurant and bar in Canggu, so we called in a favour. The venue doesn't normally host weddings, but they made an exception for us. They planned the wedding for us, then Paul threw a party for them. We locked in the date, 20 February 2020, and started counting down the days.

My family was especially excited because I was the first grandchild to get married. My grandma, who I've always been close with, was adamant she would be there. She was seventy-eight, but nothing was going to keep her from seeing me walk down the aisle. Poppa sadly had issues with deep vein thrombosis, so he wasn't able to travel.

We asked Brett to be the officiant. He loved it because for the first time, we were organising him, instead of the other way around. We'd planned everything down to the finest detail. We arrived in Bali a week before the wedding and Paul enjoyed his version of a bucks' party. The boys surfed, trained and got healthy for the festivities ahead. Meanwhile, my bridesmaids – including my sisters, Laura, Ellidy, Corey, Gita and Emma – threw me a hens' party in Sydney before we flew over to Bali for 'The Festival of Fisher'.

The sun shone bright on our big day. I wore a custom Grace Loves Lace gown and Paul was dapper in a cream suit. Just before the boys left their hotel to head to The Lawn, Brett took a photo of Paul. He'd never seen him so nervous or 'in the zone'. It was such a moment in time, the space between going from a partner to a husband. I'd never been more ready for anything.

Walking down the aisle and seeing Paul there waiting for me, I felt like I was floating. Paul later told me how special that moment was for him. 'You were just so beautiful, it was mind-blowing. Seeing you walk down the aisle was the pinnacle of the whole day for me,' he says now.

I cried as Paul read his vows: 'You are my soulmate and my best friend, and I am so glad we found each other. I pinch myself every day how lucky I am to have you in my life. I love you Chloe, and I'm so proud to call you my wife.'

I was a wife. Paul's wife. It was the best feeling in the world. We had a private moment together in the back of the car on our way to getting our wedding photos taken. It was just the two of us. We were drinking a glass of champagne when Paul told me to stay still. He pulled out his phone and took a photo of me. He wanted to remember that moment – being newly married to the love of his life – forever. That photo is the one he looks back on the most now.

We rushed through the professional photos so we could get to the party. When we walked into the reception as Mr and Mrs Fisher – to the soundtrack of Cher's 'Believe' – Paul tried to twirl me, and I promptly fell face-first onto the floor. It was hilarious, and classic us.

The whole day was pure elation; the definition of cloud nine. It's impossible to choose a favourite moment. I loved Laura's cheeky maid of honour speech, Ellidy's wedding cake demolition, Chumpy's epic dance moves, and – more than anything – my grandma's joyous smile. I couldn't have asked for a better day. We partied well into the night, and I really let my hair down. Normally it's Paul who goes a bit overboard, but I definitely took the cake on our wedding day.

I woke up the next day with a sore head – and a husband! It was the first day of the rest of our lives. We were stupidly happy – and blissfully naïve. We had no fucking idea what the universe had in store for us.

Six days after our wedding, we were still riding the high and celebrating with friends at Desa Potato Head. My mum called me to tell me Grandma – who was staying in Legian with my aunty and cousins – was having trouble breathing. She had underlying respiratory issues, so it was a concern.

Everyone was getting increasingly worried, and the family booked Grandma a seat on the next available flight home later that night. However, things escalated, and Grandma went downhill fast.

My mum called me again. 'Grandma's really not well,' she said. 'We've called an ambulance. I think you should meet us at the hospital.'

The ambulance took hours to arrive. When it finally did, Grandma was in a bad way. She desperately needed oxygen to help with her breathing, but the oxygen system in the ambulance was faulty and didn't work.

I rushed to the hospital. We still didn't know how serious things were, so Paul didn't even come with me. He stayed by the pool with our mates. In the car on the way to the hospital, a wave of dread washed over me. I looked at the clock and saw it was 11.11 am. I made a silent wish: *Please be okay, Grandma, please.*

I arrived at the hospital with my sisters just as the ambulance was pulling up. Mum was still stuck in traffic coming from Canggu. I'll never forget the moment the ambulance doors opened and I saw my grandma. *Oh my fucking God, this is over,* I thought to myself.

I'd never seen anything like it. Grandma's whole body had swollen up like a balloon. Her eyes were closed and she was unresponsive. When they took her into a hospital room, I could barely be in the room with her. I'm so grateful my sister Olivia, who's a nurse, was there. It was Liv who felt for a pulse in the hospital room. She couldn't find one. Still, the medical team continued to perform CPR.

I called Paul straight away. 'Hey, you really need to get here. This isn't good,' I told him.

I was watching the doctors push down on my grandmother's chest when I heard a crack, which I assumed was them breaking one of her ribs. Then I noticed the blood. It was coming out of her mouth. It was too late. She was gone.

Grandma had passed away before she even got to the hospital. She died in the ambulance on the way there. I'm certain she left the world at the exact moment my stomach sank on the drive there, at 11.11 am.

The grief was excruciating. So was the guilt. My beautiful grandma passed away in a foreign country attending *my* wedding. I blamed myself. 'She would still be alive if she was in Australia,' I told myself.

The last photo we have of Grandma is her holding a bunch of white roses at my wedding.

When Mum eventually made it to the hospital, she had to see her mother's lifeless body. My brother – who was the only one of us back in Sydney – and our uncle had to go over to Pop's house and tell him Grandma wasn't coming home that night.

Pop was inconsolable. 'I should've been there for her,' he cried to Cooper. 'I'll never forgive myself, mate. Never.'

The fallout was devastating. My mum's family were never the same again.

My aunties and uncles left Bali to go back to Australia, but my parents, siblings, Paul and I stayed to organise the logistics of getting Grandma home.

The day after Grandma's passing, we held a Balinese ceremony to set her spirit free. On the shore at Seminyak Beach, we made traditional offerings – canang sari – to the gods. We wore marigold flower chains around our necks and received a water blessing from a local woman, then sat in the sand next to each other and cried. Paul was by my side the whole time. He held me together when I was sure I would crack into a million pieces under the weight of my sadness.

I got 11:11 tattooed on my wrist and a rose on the back of my arm, in honour of my grandma.

Returning to Australia was an emotional ride. We'd gone from the dizzying high of our wedding to the devastating loss of my grandma in the space of a week. As if that wasn't enough, a virus outbreak erupted at the same time. The turmoil was relentless. While we were organising the repatriation of Grandma's body at the very start of March 2020, we heard talk of international borders closing because of the coronavirus. That added an extra layer of pressure to an already hard time.

We weren't the only ones feeling the strain. It was a strange time for absolutely everyone. It felt like a line was drawn in drying concrete. On one side was life before the pandemic, and on the other was after. For me, there were two other lines next to that one, marking life before marriage and life before losing my grandma. That last line wasn't straight – it was jagged, like the edges of a broken heart.

We flew back to Sydney on the same plane as Grandma's body. The family had planned a funeral at Mona Vale Sacred Heart Church. The place was packed to the rafters with Grandma's family and friends – she was so loved – and it was a beautiful ceremony, albeit very solemn. Seeing my pop was the hardest thing. I didn't know what to say. He was so, *so* sad. Poppa and Grandma had been together all of their lives; they were married for fifty-odd years. He lost a piece of himself with her. I don't think he blamed me for what happened, but I still struggle with the guilt. He didn't get to say goodbye to his soulmate or tell her he loved her one last time. He thought she was coming home early; instead, she didn't come home at all. It was so unfair.

I remember looking at Pop sitting in his sadness and thinking, *There's nothing I can do to make this better.* As soon as I had that thought, I had another: *The only thing that might help is if I have a baby. If Poppa gets to meet my baby, he'll be able to tell Grandma all about them when he joins her one day.*

A gentle reminder

Grief is not linear, and healing has no timeline.

Four

UNCHARTED TERRITORY

First comes love, then comes marriage, then comes baby in a golden carriage. That was the order of things; we'd been taught as much as little kids learning nursery rhymes at preschool. At our wedding, I openly told people we were going to start trying for a baby straight away. It was the obvious next step.

In saying that, even before we were married, we'd never been careful. I was on the pill from age sixteen to twenty-five, but I came off it once Paul and I had been together a while. After that, we were pretty lax about contraception. There was no question that if I accidentally fell pregnant, we would have the baby. Considering how carefree we were, it might have been surprising that we hadn't already had an accident, but I didn't think about that at the time. I figured it would happen when it was meant to happen, and I hoped that would be after we got married.

When we returned to Sydney after Bali, I went to see an acupuncturist for people wanting to fall pregnant, who came highly recommended. I'd had acupuncture before and was a big fan. At the appointment, I explained that I was hoping to have a baby. 'Great. Let's get your bloods done today so we know where you're at. Then we can figure out what program to start you on,' the acupuncturist said. 'I'll email you when we get the results and book in for another appointment.'

While I was waiting for the results of my blood test, the world was waiting to see what was going to happen with coronavirus. Everything was uncertain. Paul had gigs booked in the States, and we had planned to head back to LA in March, but the virus threw a spanner in the works. Things started getting cancelled: gigs, flights, selective hospital procedures. Paul had a number of phone calls with his management team, but the conversations went around in circles. Should we come? Should we stay? Should we come? Should we stay? No-one had any answers. 'The shows are still on, and I'm not going to be the one to pull the pin. I'm not going to let down the fans,' Paul rationalised.

We were optimistic, so we stuck with our plan to go to the States, and took the mandatory Covid test twenty-four hours before our flight. It was such a weird time to travel.

It felt like the world was on the brink of something: chaos, calamity, a cliff face.

The day we arrived in LA, we both went to Paul's management office to check in with the team. Paul was chatting to Brett, and I was going through my emails. For some reason, I checked my junk folder and saw an email from my doctor, who'd done the blood test for my acupuncturist. I nearly dropped my phone when I read the contents of the email.

'Did you know that you were pregnant?' the doctor wrote.

'Oh my fucking god,' I screamed, startling Paul and Brett. 'I'm pregnant!'

I was ecstatic. Paul was – in his words – 'frothing'. Brett was still alarmed at my scream, but also very happy for us.

It felt fitting. I was a honeymoon baby – my parents fell pregnant with me as newlyweds in Fiji – and now I was having my own 'honeymoon' baby. Just like the nursery rhyme prophesied, Paul and I had fallen pregnant the day after our wedding. I didn't know it at the time, but on our flight home from Bali, I'd been carrying more than my luggage.

My mum was the same. She came back from Fiji with a happy surprise – and a hell of a story. My parents' honeymoon coincided with Cyclone Sina in 1990. They spent the entire trip inside their hotel room, mostly in the bathroom, where they had to fill up the tub and sink with water for drinking. Outside, the wind roared with fury. Inside, my parents tried to make the best of the situation.

When Mum found out she was pregnant with me, she flirted with the idea of calling me Sina, in honour of the cyclone that led to my conception. Thankfully, she decided against it.

When I found out I was pregnant, I burst into happy sobs. I'd cried so many sad tears over my grandma that I didn't think I had any tears left. Once again, the moment felt bittersweet. I was overjoyed to be pregnant – it was all I'd ever wanted – but I was heartbroken that my grandma wasn't there to hear the good news. She would never meet her first great-grandchild. *At least Poppa will get to meet the baby,* I thought.

I didn't have time to process all my emotions because that very night, everything shut down. The World Health Organization declared coronavirus a pandemic. Australian travellers were encouraged to return home. American venues cancelled all upcoming gigs. The shows Paul had come over to do were no longer happening.

After a whirlwind twenty-four hours in the States, we were back on a plane to Australia. We were the first flight ordered to do home quarantine. When we landed in Sydney, we went straight to Laura's apartment in North Narrabeen, which was vacant. It was the best of times because I was so happy to be pregnant; the worst of times because I was grieving my grandma; and the weirdest of times because the entire planet was in uncharted territory. As everything else came to a standstill, I tried to focus on the baby growing inside me.

While in isolation, we video-called our closest friends and told them I was pregnant. It was weird not being able to share the news in person, but everyone was over the moon for us. Paul was especially over the moon because my boobs were huge. I had all the early pregnancy symptoms: tender (and, yes, epic) boobs, fatigue and some nausea. The morning sickness made it feel real; so did buying our first piece of baby clothing. We ordered a little brown onesie for the baby, and I couldn't believe how tiny it was. When the onesie arrived, I started picturing the baby's nursery in our brand-new house . . .

'I want to raise my kids on the Goldy.' Paul meant what he'd said. Before our wedding, we started looking at real estate in Queensland, and I got to know the area better while visiting Ellidy and Chumpy. I can't pinpoint exactly when Ell and I became close. It was sometime between our Vegas trip, my wig-themed birthday party in 2016 (where Ell wore a pastel pink number and Chumpy had a platinum blond mullet) and too many boozy lunches to count. Her being one of my bridesmaids cemented our closeness. So when Ellidy and Chumpy moved to Palm Beach on the Goldy, I felt less scared about moving to a place I'd never lived before. The thought of having friends nearby and not being totally on my own put me at ease.

Paul began to manifest his dream house. Another fun fact about Paul: he is big into manifestation. He swears he's manifested every single thing he has today, including me. He started doing it after a surf camp when he was a kid. The coach on the camp, who Paul admired a lot, told the group to manifest themselves on the podium at their next competition. 'Visualise yourself winning the surf comp, see yourself making the Australian team,' the coach instructed.

Paul was intrigued by the concept, and started writing down his hopes and dreams. For as long as I've known him, Paul has scribbled in journals and written on hotel notepads. It's almost a subconscious habit now. He doesn't realise he's doing it.

Paul wrote about wanting to live by the beach in a place with ocean views, so he wasn't surprised when we found our dream home for sale in Palm Beach. When we walked into the house, we immediately knew it was the one.

We both fell in love with the home, even though it was entirely out of our price range at the time. Paul trusted in his manifestation though. 'This is our place,' he assured me. 'I want this. I'm going to take out a huge mortgage and I'm going to work my arse off to pay for it. I'm going to provide for my family and for you, and we're going to have the best life.'

Who was I to argue with that?

Just like Paul said he would, he took out a huge mortgage and we bought the Palm Beach house of our dreams. We were moving to the Goldy, where Paul always wanted to raise his kids. The future he imagined was becoming a reality – after a long settlement period. Because of the wait, we decided to rent a little place in Currumbin for the few months before we could move into our new home. The rental was a literal treehouse, with snakes in the rafters and bush all around us. It was such a cool spot, and I was happy to be settled somewhere, even temporarily.

I was keen to book in for an ultrasound as soon as I could, but it was surprisingly hard to make an appointment. I don't know whether it was because I was still early in my pregnancy, because Covid was impacting bookings or because I was new to the area, but I couldn't get in for a scan for a couple of weeks. I went to a GP, who ordered another blood test. My hCG levels confirmed I was pregnant.

I was giddy with excitement at the thought of seeing our baby for the first time. The only downside was that I had to go to the ultrasound appointment alone because of restrictions. Paul sat impatiently in the waiting room.

Not long after the scan started, my giddiness went from excitement to nerves. The ultrasound technician was wearing a mask, but I could tell from her body language that something wasn't right. 'I'm sorry, we can't see a heartbeat in the sac,' the tech eventually explained. 'It's only measuring quite small, so you might not be as far along as you think.'

That didn't sit well with me. I knew exactly how far along I was because I knew when I'd had my last period. My GP said we'd need to wait two weeks, then do another scan to see if the baby had grown. I sensed something was wrong.

Paul and I spent the night googling 'gestational sac', 'ectopic pregnancy' and 'signs of a miscarriage'. The next fortnight was pure hell. I kept hoping that something would change. I prayed that they'd made a mistake, that it was all a big misunderstanding. It wasn't.

At the second ultrasound, the tech didn't say anything. She didn't even show me the screen. It was awful.

My GP confirmed that I'd had a miscarriage. The baby was gone. I knew it before she said the words. The ultrasound tech's silence had spoken louder than any words could.

'It's likely that the baby implanted in the fallopian tube rather than the sac, which caused the miscarriage,' the GP explained.

My first thought was, *What the fuck*. I couldn't believe I'd had a miscarriage. Naïvely, I didn't think it was something that would happen to me. I was *twenty-eight*. I wrongly thought I was too young to lose a baby. That was something that happened to older women. Other women. Not me.

I couldn't stop the tears. 'Why is this happening to me? What did I do wrong?' I asked.

'This is very common, it happens to one in four pregnancies,' the GP explained.

On a surface level, I knew miscarriages were common. I even knew my mum had had one – not that we ever spoke about it – but I'd never imagined it was something I would experience. Fuck, I was clueless.

The GP ran through my options. I could wait for the loss to happen naturally, I could take a pill to make it happen medically, or I could have a D&C. I booked in to have a D&C the next day. I wanted to flush everything out so I could try again.

Before the surgery, I took two tablets to soften my uterus. The medication induced mini-contractions, which were incredibly painful. I was thankful when they put me under anaesthetic and knocked me out. I went into that surgery whole, and I came out with a piece of me missing. When I woke up in hospital with compression socks on my feet, I couldn't stop crying. I went home feeling empty.

I sent a copy-and-paste text to the friends who'd known I was pregnant, telling them I'd had a miscarriage and would reach out when I was ready to talk. I had no words. I found it really hard to talk about the loss, so I didn't. Instead, I shut off completely. Still, my OGs Laura, Ellidy and my close friend Renee would rock up on my doorstep with food, ice cream and cuddles. Lots of people sent flowers; my sister Olivia bought me the most beautiful orchid with a white flower speckled with splashes of purple. Our friends' daughter Scout made us a card that said, 'Dear Fish and Chloe, I am very sorry about your baby, but I really hope you're okay.' She drew me as a bird with orange feathers.

Feathers, always feathers.

It was right after the D&C, when I was still struggling to talk about the miscarriage in real life, that I posted a message on Instagram. I bared my soul: *This past week we should have been 9.5 weeks pregnant, both completely and utterly in love and over the moon, something that I've dreamed about my whole life, my little miracle that was conceived right between our wedding and the death of my beautiful grandma in Bali.*

On April 17, I said goodbye to you, my first real baby, and although I will never get to hold you in my arms, your daddy and I will hold you in our hearts forever and ever, I continued. *Rest easy our little Fish. Lucky Grandma, the first one to meet you.*

I wanted to start trying for another baby straight away. The GP recommended we wait at least six weeks, or until after my next period, which felt like a waste of a month. My life began to revolve around my menstrual cycle.

I wasn't the only one. After we moved into our Palm Beach home, I had Ellidy and Chumpy over one night for dinner. Paul was away, so it was just the three of us, sitting around the table, joking, laughing and carrying on. We were all pretty tipsy. 'You guys are such fools,' Chumpy teased. That's why we got on so well.

I knew Ell and Chump had been trying to fall pregnant for a while, but they hadn't had any luck yet. That night, while we were having dinner, Ell got a call from her doctor. She'd gone in for an Anti-Mullerian Hormone (AMH) test to find out how many eggs she had. The doctor called with bad news. Ell had a low egg count, which might explain why she hadn't conceived yet. 'Don't be alarmed,' the doctor tried to reassure her. 'It could just mean getting pregnant might be a little bit more difficult for you.'

Ell was understandably gutted. I knew how she felt. We both drowned our sorrows that night.

I'll admit, I'd never heard of an AMH test before that night. At that point in my journey, I felt clueless about fertility. As teenagers, we were never taught about conceiving; it was all about contraception. Our sex ed classes purely focused on how not to get pregnant. No-one mentioned how hard it actually is to get pregnant – so many stars need to align. The ovary needs to release an egg, the egg needs to be fertilised by sperm, the fertilised egg needs to travel down the fallopian tube to the uterus, the embryo needs to attach to the lining of the uterus. And that's just the very beginning.

Having a baby may be the most natural thing in the world, but that doesn't mean it's easy. Nature, luck, timing, chance and sometimes science all play a part. I was learning the hard way that conception was the one thing I couldn't control. I had always been organised and driven, but I couldn't spreadsheet my way to a baby. As each month passed, and my period inevitably came, I became more and more frustrated with the lack of control.

I tried to focus on the things I could control, and to distract myself from only thinking about becoming a mum. I had sold Aloé Swimwear in 2019 after building it from the ground up and learning every aspect of running a business. I was a one-woman manufacturing, marketing, distribution, quality control and publicity machine, with help from my mum and sisters, who lovingly posted out orders from Australia. They did a lot of the heavy lifting for me because I was travelling so much, and that was the main reason I decided to sell the business. I was lucky to find an incredible buyer who saw my vision for the brand and ran with it.

Meanwhile, Paul and I were presented with a new business opportunity. A couple of guys reached out to us with a pitch: they wanted to launch seltzers in Australia, and they wanted us to be the face and driving force of the business. At that point in time, alcoholic seltzers were huge in America, but unheard of in Australia. The guys saw a gap in the market, and they wanted to be the ones to close it. We saw it too, and came on board to launch Hard Fizz in Australia.

We wrangled a team together, enlisted a number of influencers (read: our mates) to invest in and promote the brand, designed the cans, and introduced seltzers to Australia. It was incredible to walk into a bottle-o and see Hard Fizz on the shelves, mere months after the business's conception.

Turns out, I was better at conceiving businesses than babies. I desperately wished it was the other way around.

I still have the orchid my sister gave me after my first loss. It only flowers once a year. I can't help but think of my first baby whenever I see the white flower with splashes of purple.

The low down – expert info from Pink Elephants

Pink Elephants is a not-for-profit that was founded in 2016 to provide resources, information and peer support for anyone impacted by early pregnancy loss. The organisation gets its name from how if a mother elephant loses her baby, the other elephants in her community use their trunks to form a physical circle of support around her.

WHAT IS MISCARRIAGE?

A miscarriage is the loss of a pregnancy before twenty weeks gestation. Sadly, miscarriages are a common occurrence, with one in four pregnancies ending in loss before twenty weeks.

The term 'recurrent miscarriage' is used when women experience two or more early pregnancy losses. This affects up to five per cent of couples.

There are several different types of miscarriage:

Chemical pregnancy: A very early miscarriage that normally occurs before five weeks.

Missed miscarriage: This is where the baby has died or failed to develop but is still in your uterus, giving you no reason to believe that anything is wrong. A missed miscarriage is usually not diagnosed until a routine scan. You may still feel pregnant, or your pregnancy symptoms may have begun to subside.

Incomplete miscarriage: When some but not all of the pregnancy tissue is miscarried. You may have pain and heavy bleeding that does not subside. In some instances, a D&C will be required to remove the remaining pregnancy tissue.

Blighted ovum: Where no embryo can be detected in the uterus. A blighted ovum is usually not discovered until an early ultrasound, and it generally means that an embryo was conceived, hence a pregnancy sac was formed, but it did not develop and was reabsorbed into the wall of the uterus.

SYMPTOMS

The most common signs of miscarriage are heavy bleeding, perhaps with blood clots, and strong period-type pains. Sometimes, however, a miscarriage can occur without any symptoms at all.

In general, it is best to see your healthcare professional if any of the following symptoms occur:

- vaginal bleeding or spotting
- dull lower back pain/pressure
- cramping
- changes to vaginal discharge.

CAUSES

There are a number of possible reasons that a miscarriage may occur, but even with testing, a medical explanation is often not discovered. The most common causes can include:

- chromosomal abnormalities
- balanced translocations
- uterine abnormalities
- blood clotting disorder

- autoimmune disorders
- hormonal issues
- maternal age.

It is important to know there is nothing you could have done to prevent this – it is not your fault – and the good news is that most women who experience miscarriage will go on to have a subsequent healthy pregnancy.

TREATMENTS AND PROCEDURES

When a miscarriage has been confirmed with an ultrasound, you have options on what to do next.

An expectant/natural miscarriage: When you wait for the pregnancy to miscarry.

Dilation & curettage: A D&C is a common course of treatment for miscarriages, especially when the pregnancy is eight+ weeks. It is a fairly simple day surgery procedure that takes around twenty minutes all up, though you will be required to stay at the hospital for four to five hours, including time in recovery. The D&C is performed under a light general anaesthetic. The doctor will remove the contents in your uterus while also scraping away the uterine lining. Your doctor will be able to send the tissue with your baby for testing if you wish.

Medical management: If you would prefer not to have a D&C, but do not want to wait with uncertainty for your miscarriage to occur naturally, you can opt to take medication that will induce the body to expel the pregnancy.

The most commonly used medication is called Misoprostol, which has been proven to be effective for approximately eighty per cent of women whose miscarriages occur before nine weeks. It can be administered vaginally or orally, taking one dose per day for two consecutive days.

Five

GONE TOO SOON

It was a rare occasion. Paul and Chumpy were in town at the same time. Before the pandemic, they'd both been travelling so much, it was hard to get them in the same time zone, let alone the same room. We jumped at the chance to get the whole gang together and headed over to Ell and Chump's place for dinner. Fish tacos were on the menu, because Chump had caught some fresh reef fish. He'd been getting really into spearfishing since moving to Palm Beach.

'You should come out with me tomorrow,' Chumpy suggested to Paul.

'Nah, thanks mate. Don't be fooled by the name, I'm not a fisherman,' Paul joked. 'And I'm not keen on being shark bait out on the reef.'

Still, we were more than happy to eat the spoils of Chumpy's spearfishing haul. Over a delightful bottle of red wine, I chatted to Chumpy about wanting to buy a new car. I'd never owned a new car in my life, and I was worried it was too extravagant.

'It's just so much money,' I said.

That's when Chump said something profound. 'You don't die with money, Chlo,' he reminded me. 'You guys have worked so hard, buy the fucking car, you deserve it.'

He was right, of course he was. Chumpy was wise beyond his years and had such a presence about him. He was the life of every party, the brightest spark in every room. I loved seeing him and Ell together, and we were about to see much more of them. Our new home at Palm Beach was a six-minute drive from their place. We were basically neighbours!

Ell and Chump were at the same stage in life as us, and it felt good to have them by our side. I was sure we were going to have kids at the same time and raise them together as little surfers on the Goldy.

I'll never forget that Tuesday night of fish tacos, red wine and crappy jokes. It was one of those moments in life when I thought, *Fuck, I'm so lucky.* My cheeks ached from smiling and laughing. I wanted to pinch myself; I couldn't believe this was our new normal.

Except it wasn't.

I was at lunch in Southport when I got Ell's message. *Chumpy has died,* she wrote.

You're having a laugh, I replied, thinking she was joking.

Then I called her straight away, realising she wouldn't joke about that. Dave, Ellidy's brother, answered her phone. They were at the hospital.

I didn't know what had happened, but I knew I needed to be with Ell. I jumped in the car and headed to their place, where we'd had that beautiful dinner just the night before, when Chumpy invited Paul to go spearfishing, and reminded me that you can't take money with you when you die.

Ellidy was home from the hospital by the time I arrived. She was sitting on the couch, surrounded by people, in complete shock. Ell was in the room physically, but she wasn't *there.*

I tried to piece together the unfathomable. Chumpy had gone spearfishing that morning as planned. While diving, he experienced a shallow-water blackout and drowned. A surfer found his body and dragged him to the beach – Palm Beach, metres from our house – where local lifesavers spent thirty-five minutes giving him CPR. It was no use. Chumpy was pronounced dead by paramedics at 11.15 am on 8 July 2020.

Ell had raced down to the beach after a neighbour told her someone had been pulled from the water at 19th Avenue at Palm Beach. When she pulled up there, she saw a group of people gathered on the sand. She immediately turned away.

Whatever was going on down there, she didn't want to see it. She didn't want to believe it.

My heart broke for my friend.

She was twenty-eight; too young to be a widow. He was thirty-two; too young to be gone.

More and more people turned up at Ellidy's house and rallied around her. It was Laura who first said the words 'post-mortem sperm retrieval' to me. I didn't even know that was a thing. Neither had Laura, until one of her friends lost her partner when she was thirty and pregnant with their first baby. Her friend said she wished she'd been able to retrieve her partner's sperm so she could give their baby a sibling. When Ell lost Chump, Laura immediately thought of her friend's wish.

Laura urged me to suggest the idea of sperm retrieval. 'You need to bring this up with Ell.' I'd never heard of it, and I baulked at the idea of bringing it up. I didn't think it was the time or place to talk about something like that. But Laura insisted. The conversation had to happen, and it had to happen now. Time was of the essence. In Queensland, sperm retrieval needs to happen within thirty-six hours of death, and there's a lot of red tape to cut through before it can happen.

In the end, it was Dave who had the conversation with her. As soon as he said the words 'sperm retrieval', she said, 'Yes, do it. That's what I want.'

That was all I needed. I took Ell's yes and got to work. If she wanted to go ahead with this procedure, I was going to do everything in my power to make it happen. I couldn't bring Chumpy back or soothe her aching heart, but I could wrangle doctors, lawyers and the coroner to keep her dream of having Chumpy's baby possible.

I googled every IVF clinic on the Gold Coast and started calling them one by one. 'Do you do post-mortem sperm retrieval?' I asked.

The third clinic I rang – Dr Andrew Davidson at Robina – was the first one to say yes. They could do the procedure, but we needed to find a lawyer and get the okay from the coroner before it could happen. Our friend Erika, who's a lawyer, helped with that side of things. We wrote and signed affidavits confirming Ell and Chumpy had been trying for a baby and that this was what he would have wanted, we got signed permission from Chumpy's parents because he and Ell weren't legally married, and we eventually got permission from the coroner.

We had thirty-six hours. Dr Davidson performed the sperm retrieval in the thirty-seventh hour, at 9 pm. The sample he retrieved was stored at his IVF clinic. Ell didn't even know if she would end up using it, but at least she had a choice. At least it was an option. The thought of Ell still being able to have her soulmate's child got me through some hard times.

The loss of Chumpy was enormous. He was such a loved bloke, a champion athlete, talented musician and all-round good person. Everyone who met Chumpy adored him, you couldn't help it.

Of course, it was Chumpy's family and Ell who felt the loss the most.

Just after sunrise, three days after Chumpy died, we gathered on the shore at Palm Beach. Hundreds of us paddled out to the reef where Chumpy took his last breath and formed a massive circle in the ocean. We paid tribute to our friend in the place he loved the most: the water. Ell caught a wave back into the shore, and she swears Chumpy sent it to her.

Back on the beach, we kneeled in the sand in front of the flowers that had been laid there. I sat beside Ell and held her close.

Chumpy's up there with Grandma and baby Fish. I'm glad they're together, I thought.

Ellidy wore white to Chumpy's funeral. She kept accidentally referring to it as the 'wedding' instead of the 'funeral'. That's what it should have been. Ell was young and madly in love, she should have been marrying Chumpy, not farewelling him. It was all wrong.

In the weeks and months after Chumpy's death, people handled Ellidy with care, like she was a fragile glass ornament.

I tried to treat her normally, because I knew that's what she wanted. Ell would have hated the idea of people walking on eggshells around her or being too scared to take the piss out of her. I couldn't fix things for Ell, so I focused on being there for her instead.

When Ell decided in December – five months after Chumpy's death – that she wanted to use the retrieved sperm to conceive a baby, I fully supported her choice. Some people questioned if it was too soon, if she was still too deep in the trenches of grief. But Ell wanted to get on with the future that she and Chumpy had been building together. She adopted a mantra: 'If not with you, then for you.'

A note on post-mortem sperm retrieval

In 1995, a Los Angeles man named Bruce Vernoff died unexpectedly from an allergic reaction. He was thirty. In the hours after his death, his wife Gabriela made a call that would change history. She asked Dr Cappy Rothman, director of the Center for Reproductive Medicine at Century City Hospital, if her husband's sperm could be retrieved and preserved.

The pain in Gabriela's voice convinced the doctor to perform the procedure. Thirty hours after Bruce's death, Dr Rothman and his team entered the coroner's office and extracted sperm from Bruce's epididymis, the coiled tubes behind each testis, where sperm produced in the testicles mature.

Three years later, Gabriela used the retrieved sperm to conceive a baby. Her daughter Brandalynn was born in March 1999, becoming the first child to be born from sperm collected after the father's death. Gabriela and Brandalynn paved the way for future cases.

Since 1999, post-mortem sperm retrievals (PMSRs) have been few and far between, but statistics from select sperm banks show they have increased in recent times.

The process itself is quite simple; it is performed by fertility doctors and involves making a small incision and taking out sperm cells. Most medical professionals recommend retrieving sperm within twenty-four hours of death, but sperm can potentially survive in a dead body for up to thirty-six hours.

The procedure may be simple, but the red tape is not. There is no standard legislation for harvesting a dead man's sperm, and in places where legislation exists, it varies widely. In Germany, Sweden, France and Canada, the practice is banned entirely.

In Australia, according to Dr Ben Kroon at IVF Australia, 'The law does not specifically address the issue of retrieval and use of sperm after a man's death. So, while a partner may be sure she knows what her partner "would have wanted", without supporting legal documents explicitly stating those wishes, the question of retrieval and use of sperm is not clear. In most cases, an urgent court order is needed to retrieve sperm.'

Emphasis on *urgent*. With every hour that passes after death, the chances of finding live sperm grow slimmer.

In 2012, Dr Kroon co-authored an academic article in which twenty-eight IVF clinics across Australasia were surveyed to test attitudes toward PMSR. The research found that the directors of the clinics were generally supportive of the practice, and that 'Clear, accessible and consistent law in this area would benefit medical, legal and societal stakeholders.'

In 2024, Queensland Health introduced new laws for the retrieval of gametes (reproductive cells) from deceased and unresponsive persons. For a retrieval to happen, there must be some evidence of consent. Either a person must have given their consent for the retrieval of their gametes for use by their spouse, or they must not have expressly objected to the posthumous use of their gametes and been likely to support the procedure. The 'evidence' can be text messages and emails, or recollections from loved ones about conversations with the deceased person.

Ellidy provided written statements from Chumpy's parents giving their approval, recollections from friends – including me – that they had been trying for a baby, their recent fertility appointments, and a list of baby names Ell and Chump had written together. It was what Chumpy would have wanted, and Ellidy managed to prove as much.

A 2014 US survey* found that seventy per cent of men aged eighteen to forty-four would want their spouse to be able to use their sperm after their death to have a baby, and that the presumption of consent would result in the dead men's wishes being honoured three times more often than the conservative standard of the time.

Dr Kroon, who advocates for clear guidelines around PMSR, also encourages people to discuss post-mortem sperm use in the same way we discuss organ donation.

'If couples don't have the discussion and document their wishes, it is seldom clear what one would have wanted if one dies,' he says. 'Men should consider and discuss with their partners whether they would want to father a child after their death.'

It's Ellidy's hope – and mine, too – that her story will inspire more people to have this conversation. It could be the most important chat of your life.

First post-mortem sperm retrieval baby:
https://www.latimes.com/archives/la-xpm-1999-mar-27-me-21462-story.html

* Posthumous gamete retrieval and reproduction: Would the deceased spouse consent? By Jason D. Hans, 2014, Social Science & Medicine journal *https://www.sciencedirect.com/science/article/abs/pii/S0277953614005279*

Six

SHINE

IT FELT LIKE IT WAS ME AND ELLIDY AGAINST THE WORLD. It was Ell who first introduced me to the AMH test in early 2020, and Ell who encouraged me to take one of my own at the end of the year. I'd been trying to fall pregnant naturally – taking pregnancy supplements, seeing a naturopath and doing acupuncture – for eight months without any success. Paul and I started trying to conceive again as soon as we could after our miscarriage in April. Every month, the arrival of my period felt like a failure. I didn't want to keep sitting around and waiting for it to inevitably come, so I did the AMH test to see what my egg count looked like.

The results weren't good. For someone my age, my egg count was worryingly low. At twenty-nine, I had the number of eggs equivalent to someone in their forties. It was a shock. But I was relieved to know there was a problem; I could solve a problem. That's what I'm good at. My friends don't call me Steve Jobs for nothing.

I went to my GP, who suggested IVF might be on the cards. Then I went to my naturopath, who recommended an IVF clinic in Southport. She told me Dr Kee Ong was the best in the business, and even put in a good word for me so I could get an appointment. As you can imagine, his appointments were like gold, and he was booked out for months. I didn't feel like I had months. Thanks to my naturopath, we scored an appointment with Dr Ong on 3 January 2021.

Sitting in his Southport office, he explained IVF to Paul and me in simple terms. 'Essentially, IVF uses science and nature to give you the best chance of falling pregnant,' he said. 'A woman only releases one egg a month, but with IVF, we can collect a cohort of eggs to create embryos and increase the chances of pregnancy.'

Upping our chances wasn't cheap. In 2021, a round of IVF cost $14,000, but we received a Medicare rebate of $6000. We were fortunate enough to be able to afford that. I remember someone asking me if I had a cut-off for the number of IVF rounds I was willing to undergo and pay for without success. 'No,' I replied. 'I will keep going until I have a baby.'

The first thing Dr Ong did was book me in for a laparoscopy – a type of keyhole surgery which uses a camera to see

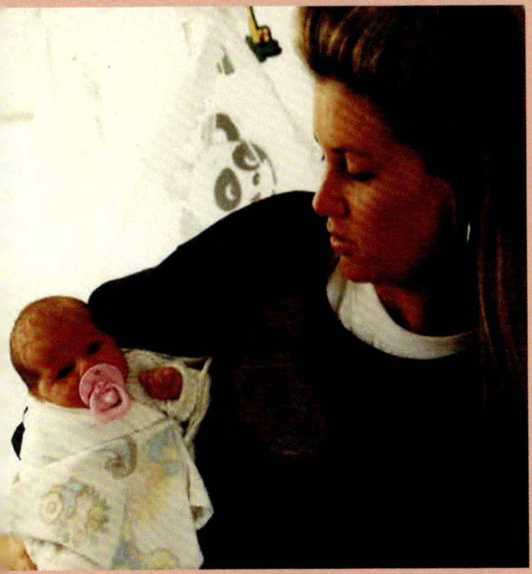

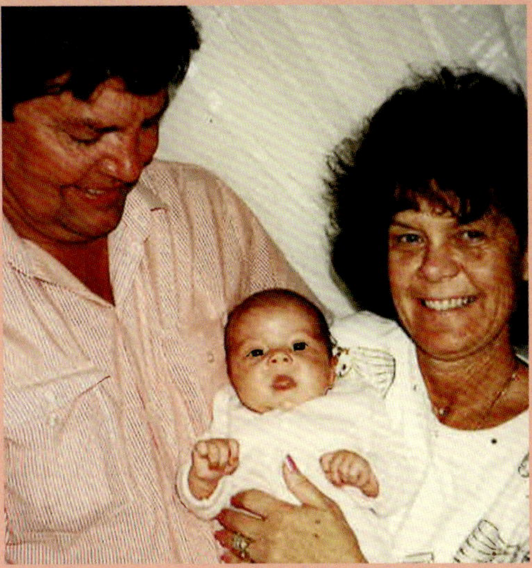

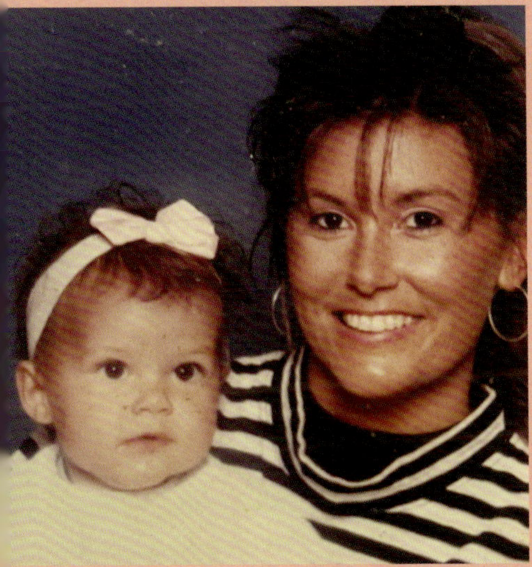

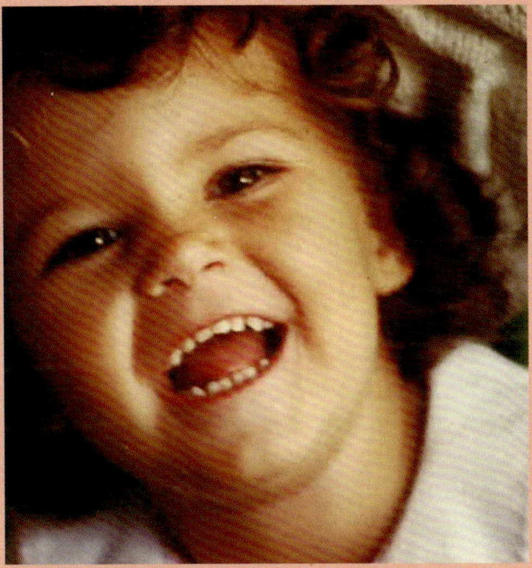

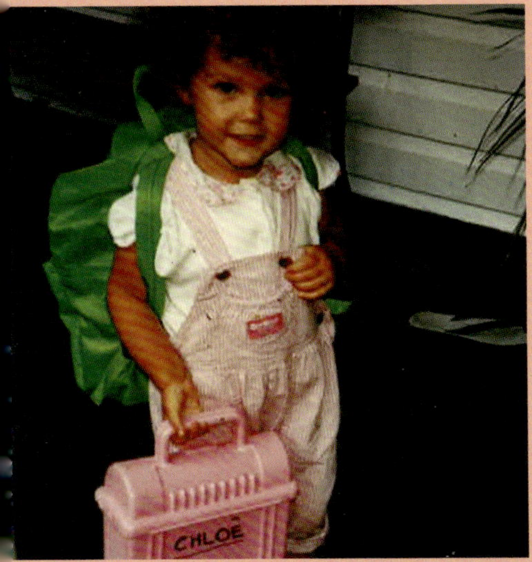
CHLOE

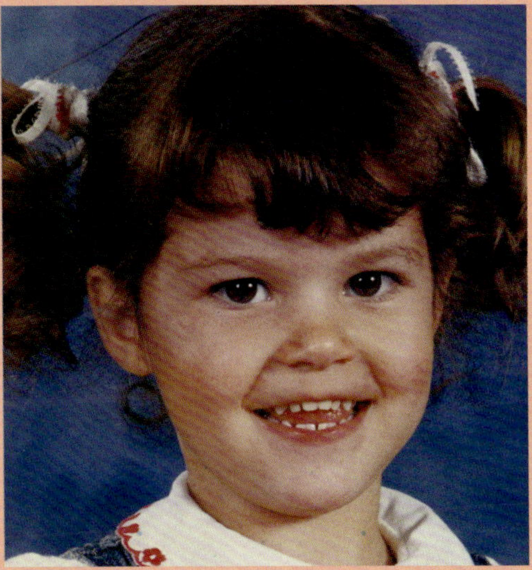

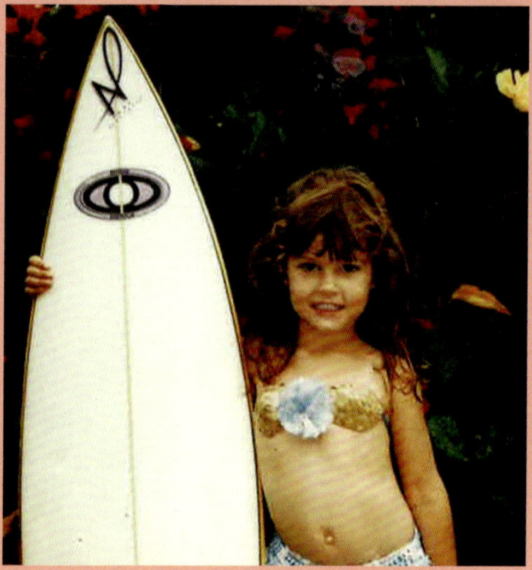

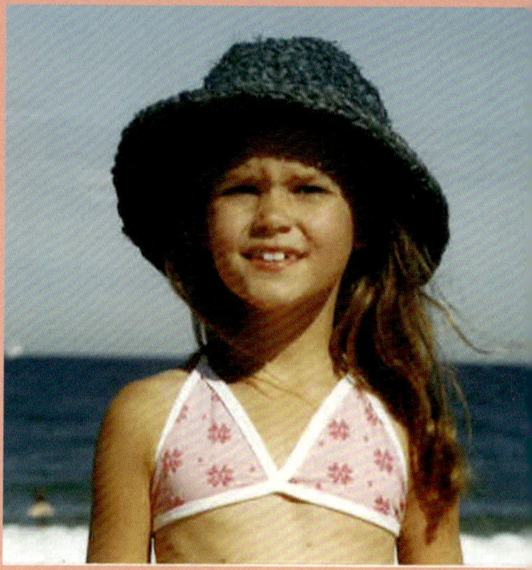

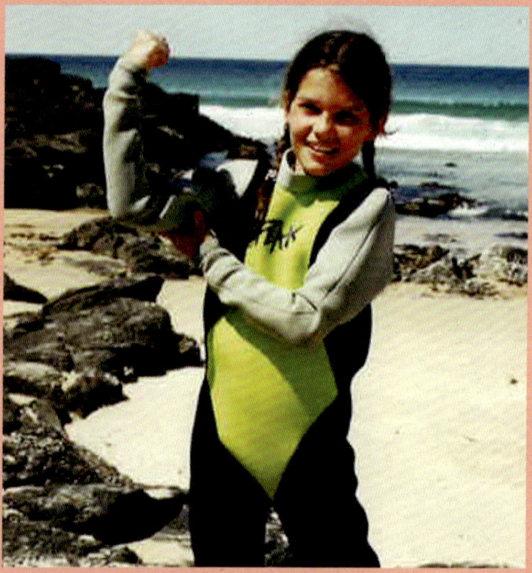

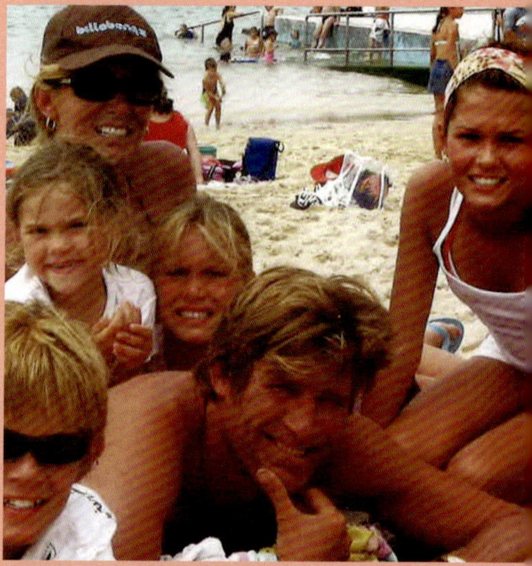

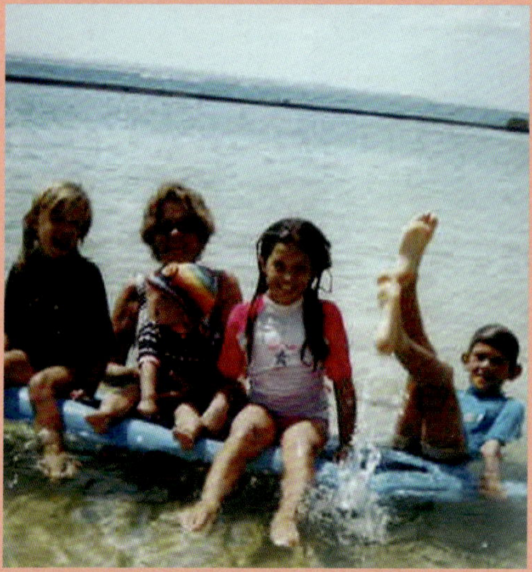

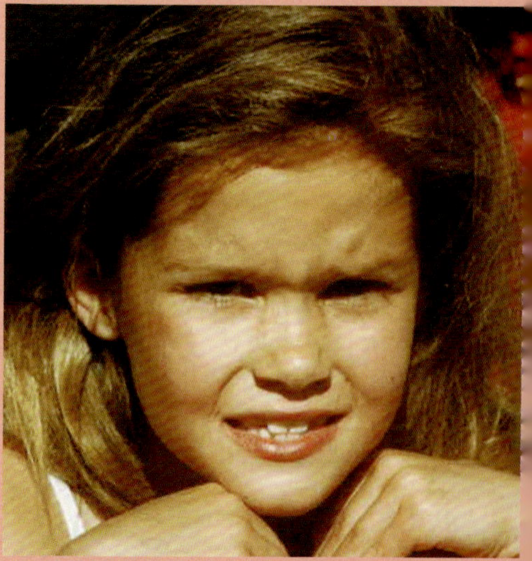

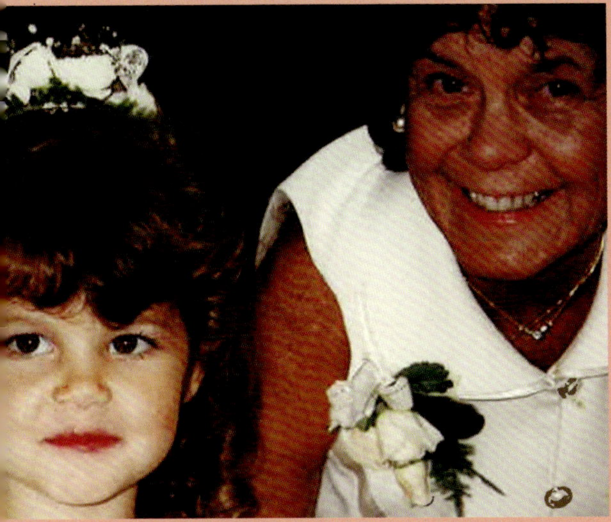
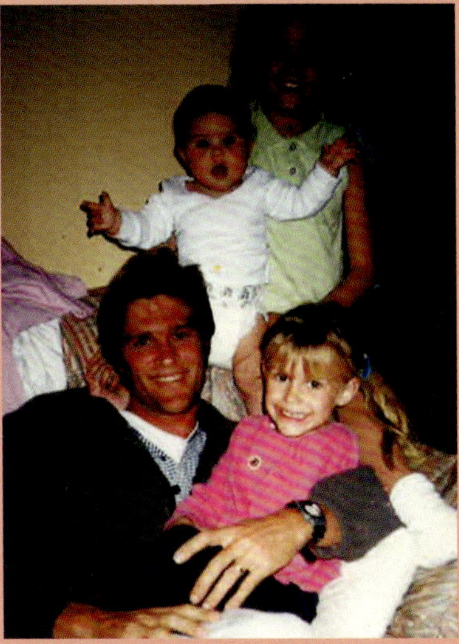
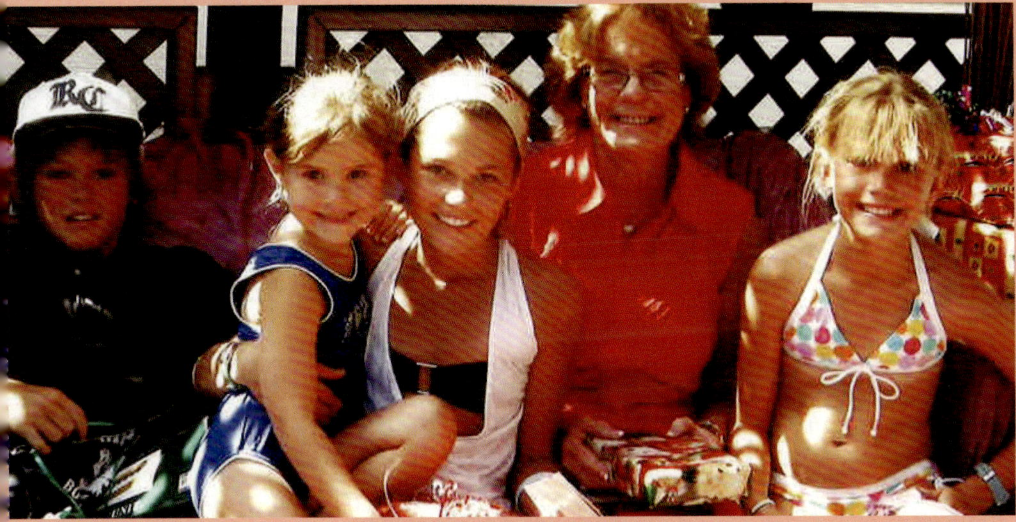
RC
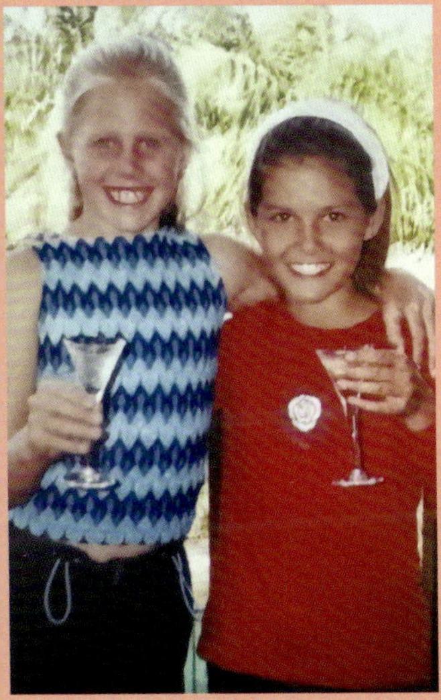
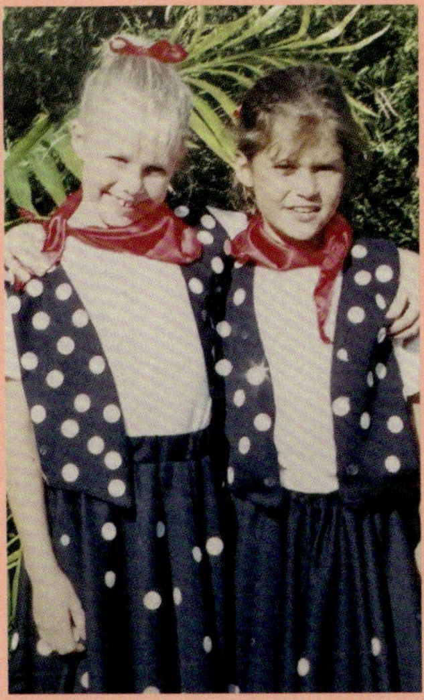
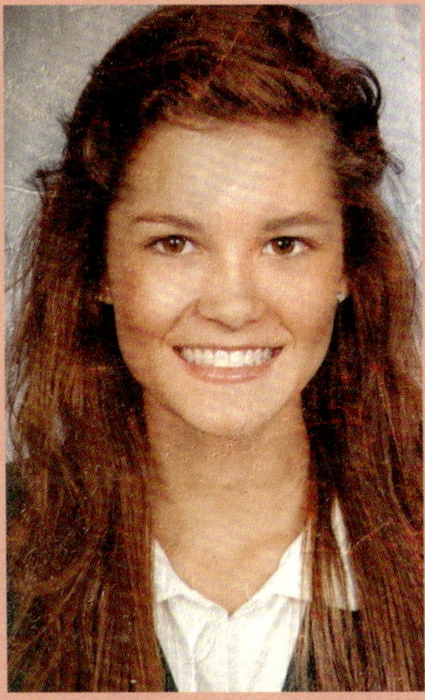

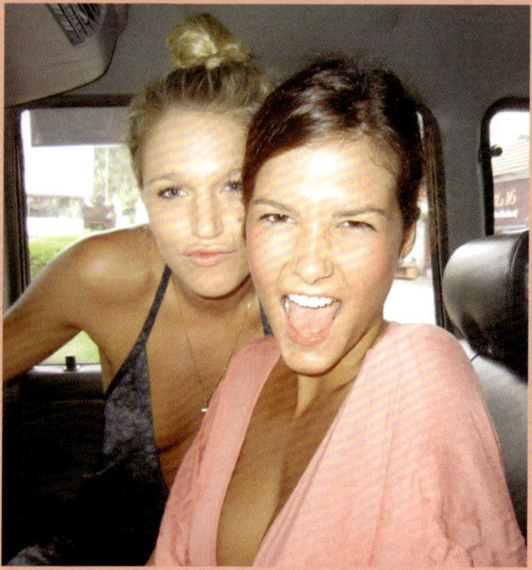
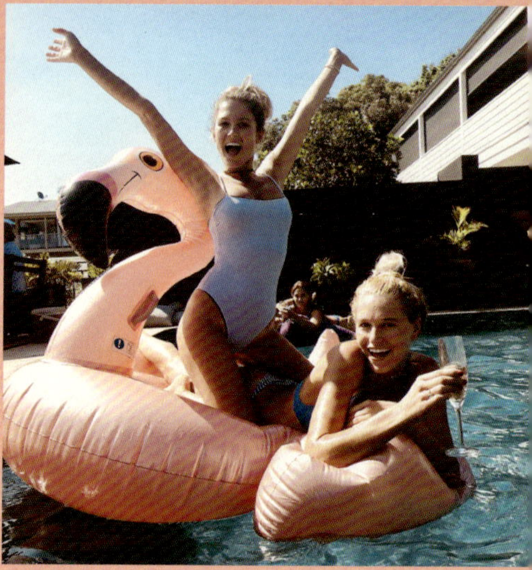
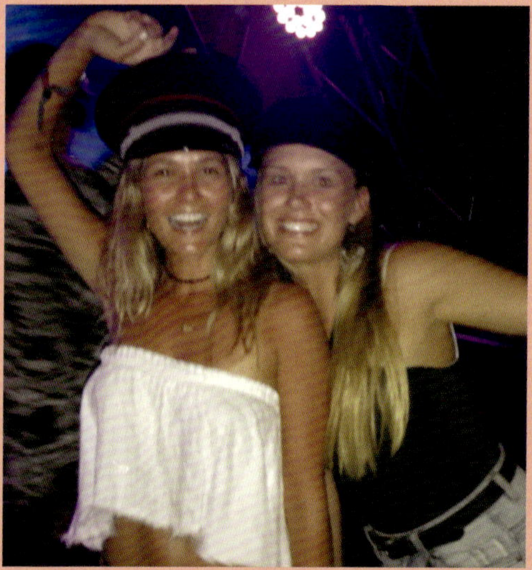
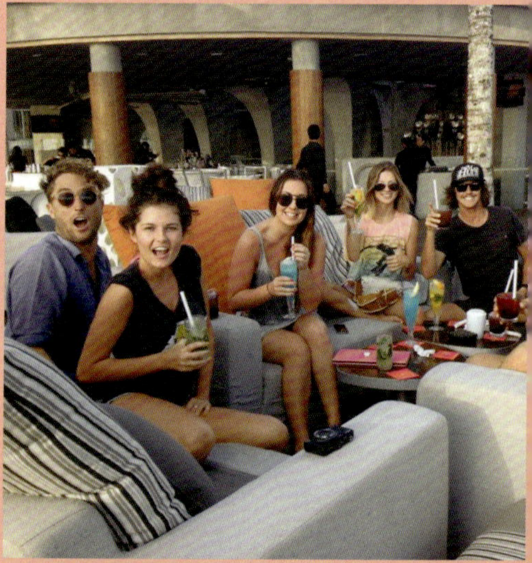
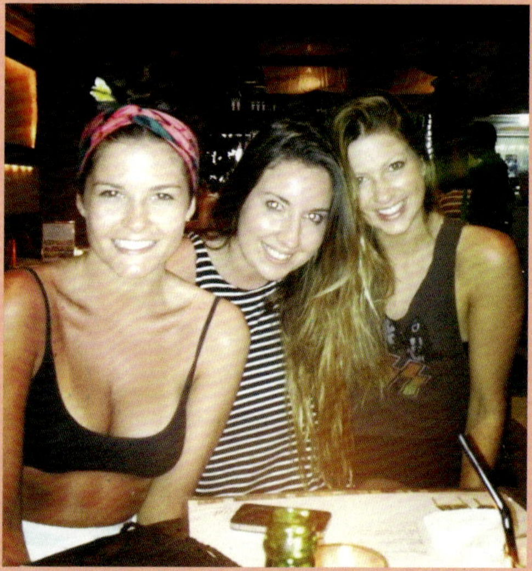
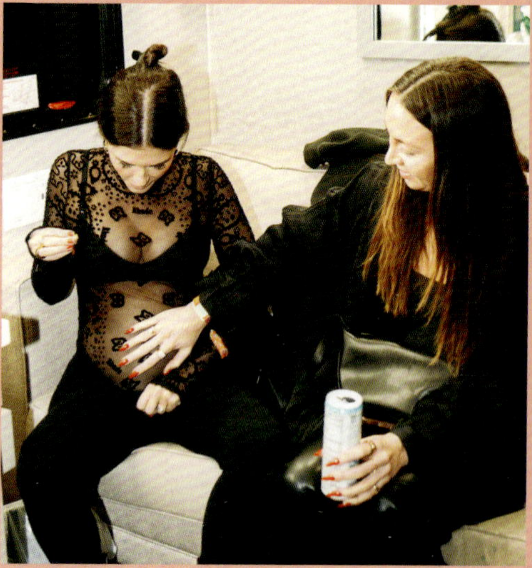

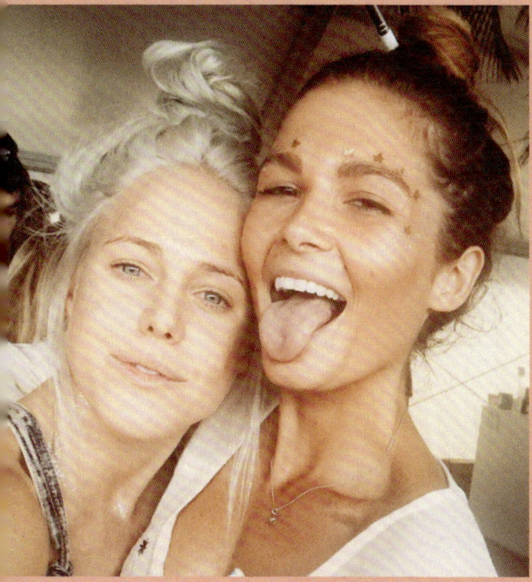

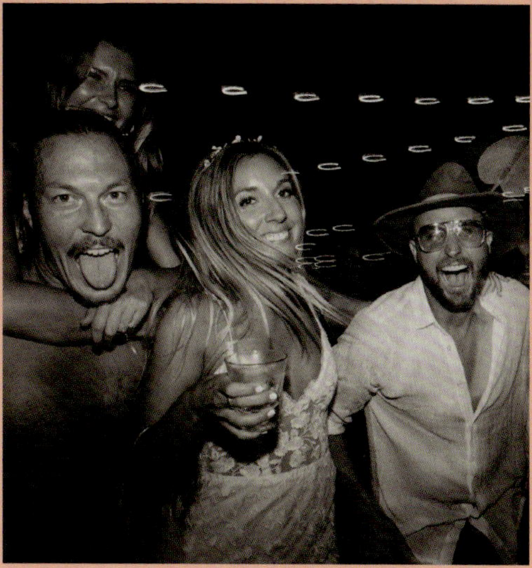

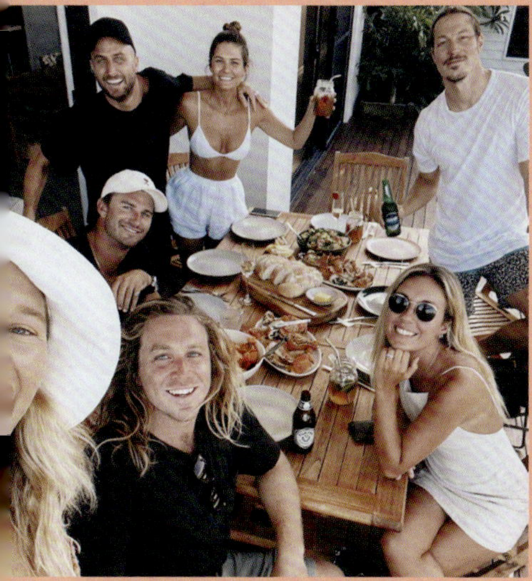

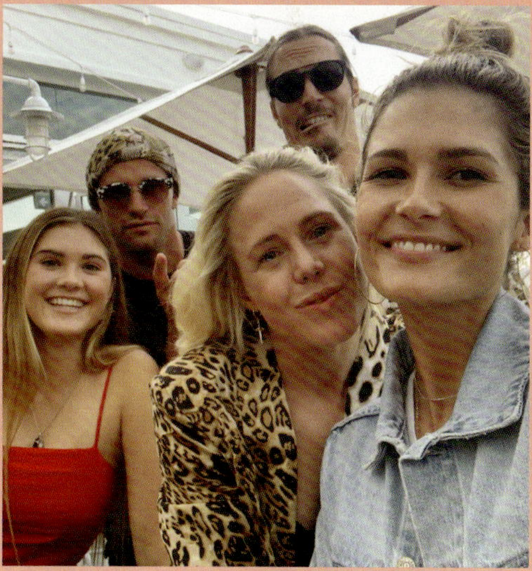

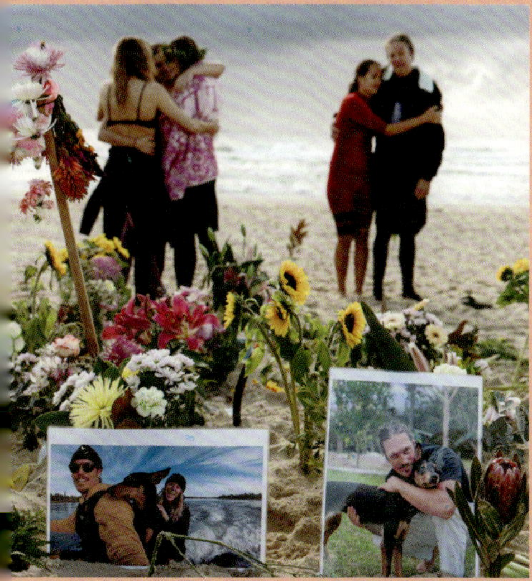

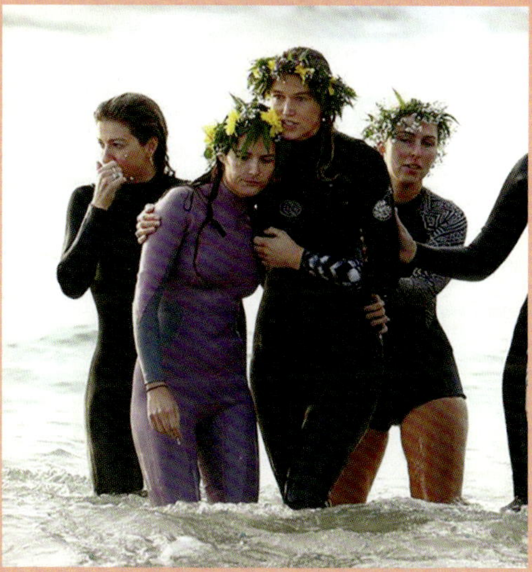

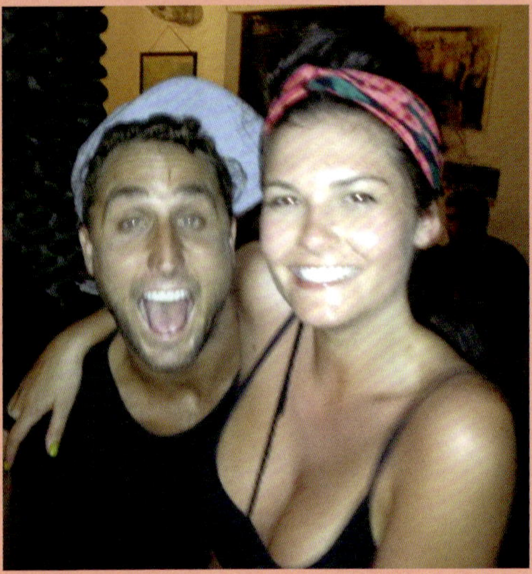

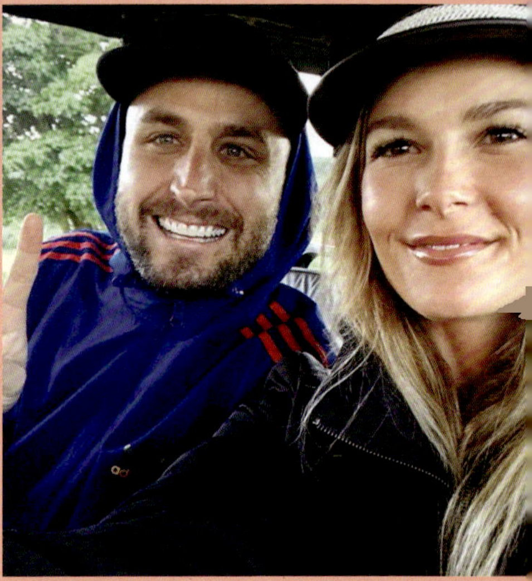

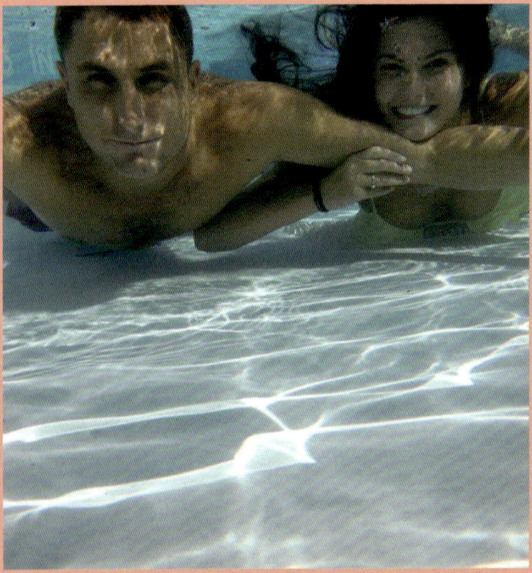

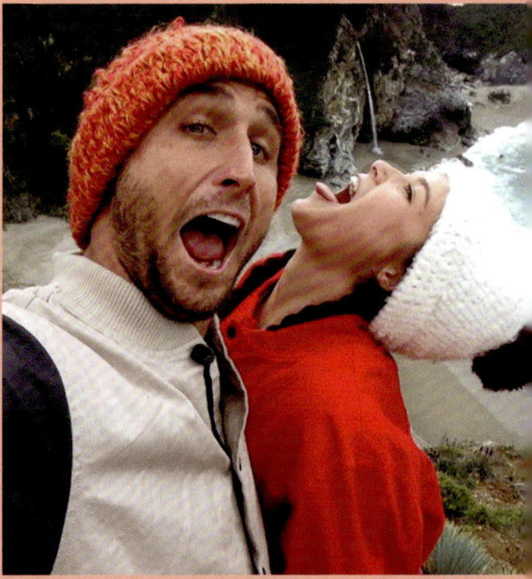

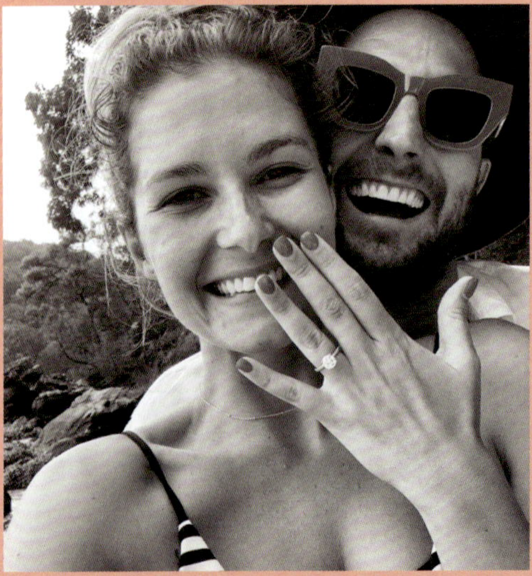

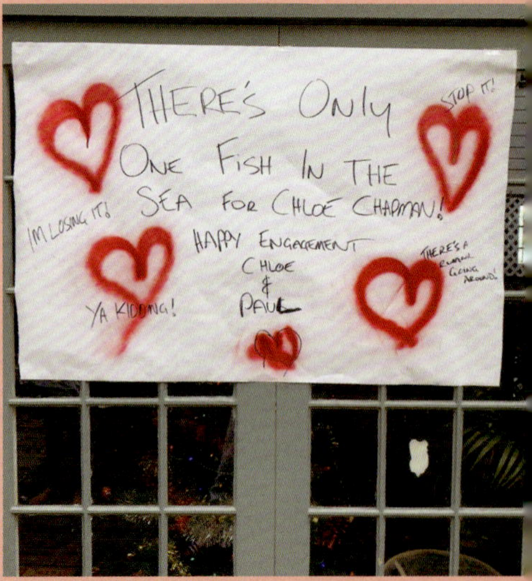
THERE'S ONLY ONE FISH IN THE SEA FOR CHLOE CHAPMAN!
STOP IT!
IM LOSING IT!
HAPPY ENGAGEMENT CHLOE & PAUL
YA KIDDING!

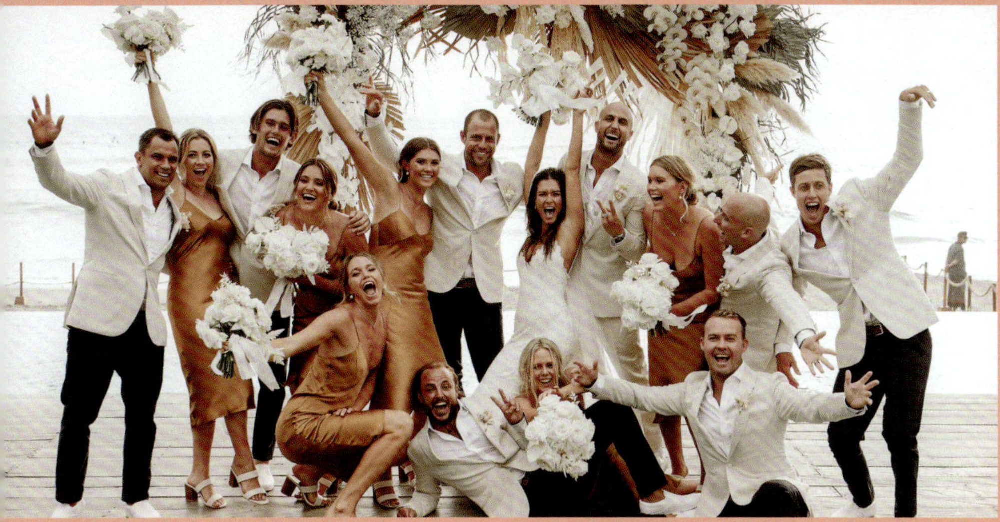

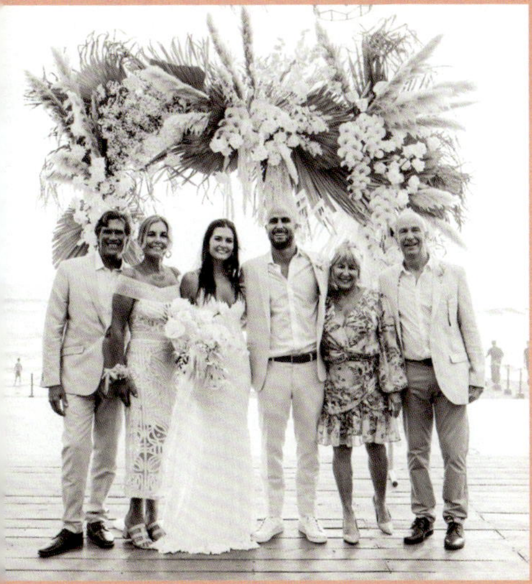

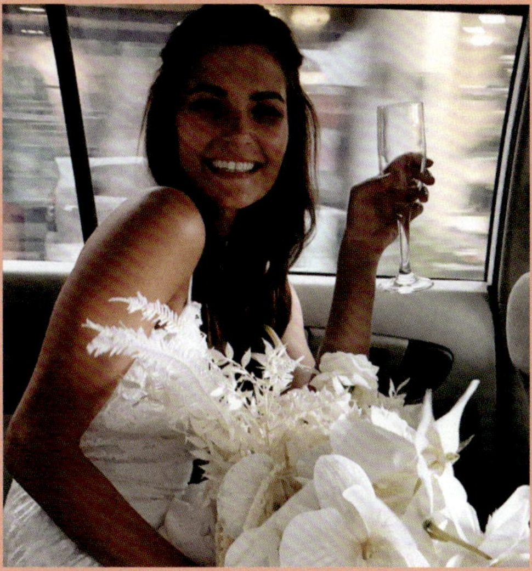

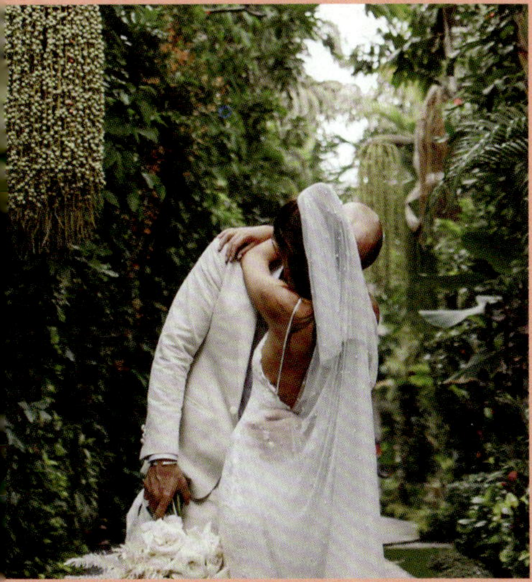

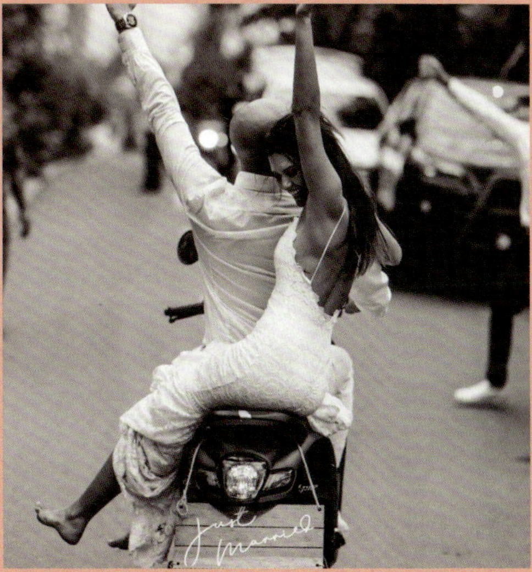
Just Married

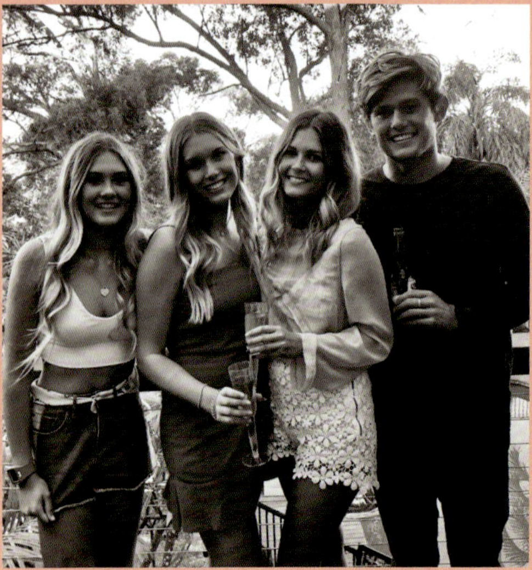
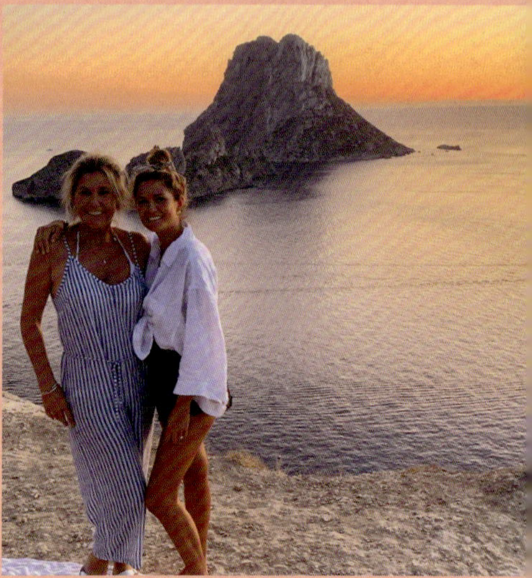
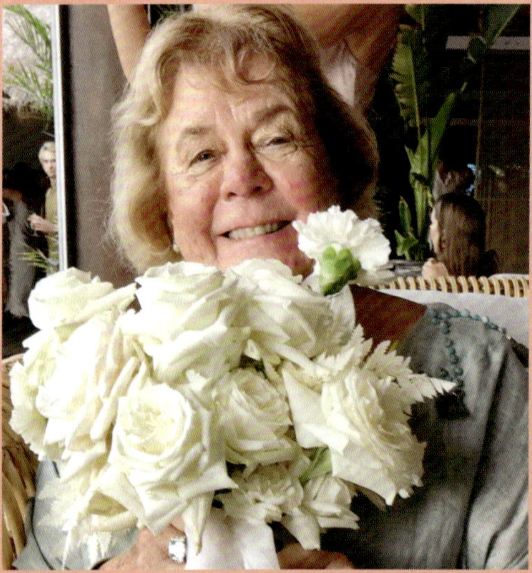
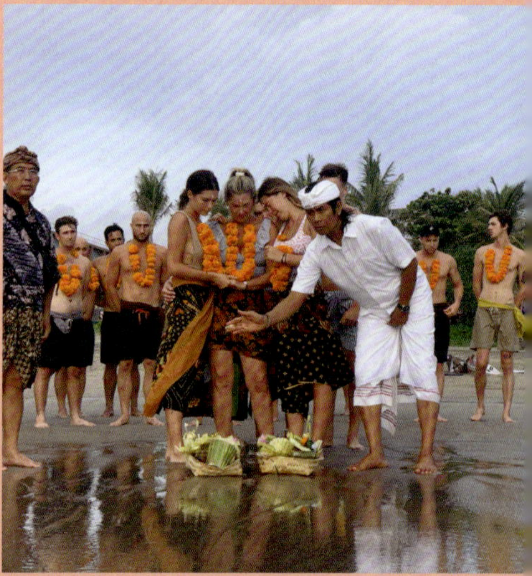
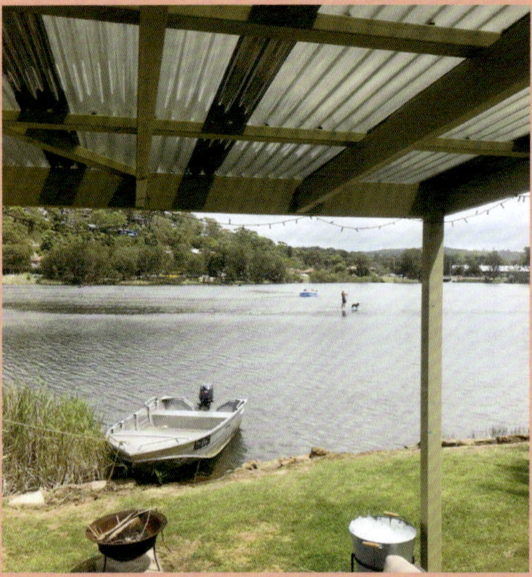
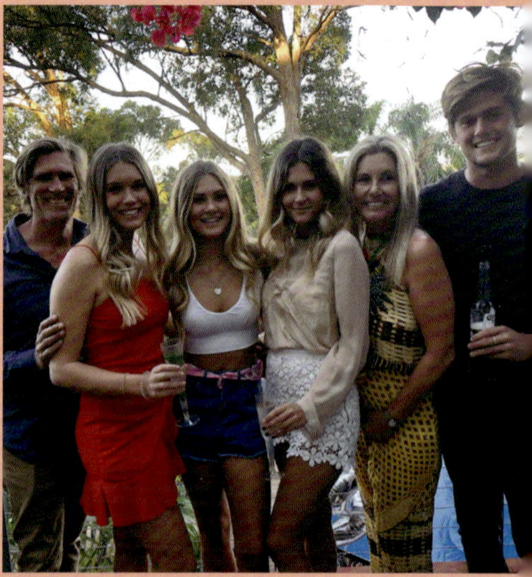

what's going on inside. While looking at my uterus, he discovered significant endometriosis, a chronic condition which occurs when tissue grows outside of the uterus.

It was a surprise to me. I'd always had regular periods, like clockwork, without any severe pain or cramping. I didn't have any of the main symptoms of endo, which can include pelvic pain and heavy and irregular periods. But I did have one symptom: I was struggling to fall pregnant.

When Dr Ong removed the endometriosis, I figured it would solve all our issues. My uterus was a clean slate, ready to go. Giddy-up. I started my first round of IVF right away, and was excited to be doing so. On day three of my next period, I began injecting myself with the prescribed medication. We videoed my first ever injection, and the footage shows my hands shaking as I press the needle into my tummy. I squealed at the sting, but smiled at Paul behind the camera afterward.

Because of my AMH level, I was on a high dose of medication, which I had to inject twice each morning and once at night. The injections include follicle stimulating hormone (FSH), luteinising hormone (LH), human chorionic gonadotropin (hCG), and gonadotropin-releasing hormone (GnRH). In English: hormones to stimulate the ovaries to produce more than one egg.

Halfway through my two weeks of injections, I went in for a scan to see how my follicles – where the eggs grow – were looking. They saw five follicles, which would hopefully translate to five eggs. At my egg retrieval procedure a week later, I was told I would be put under anaesthetic and the team would write the number of eggs they collected on my hand after the surgery. When I woke up, all groggy and disoriented, the first thing I did was look at my hand. Five. They'd gotten five eggs. I promptly burst into tears. I was so happy. That felt like a good number to me, but when I looked over at the woman sitting across from me, she had 'thirty' written on her hand.

All five of my eggs were mature, so all five were fertilised that day. That morning, Paul had visited the 'fun room' in the clinic to provide a sperm sample. He swore it was the most awkward thing he'd ever done. There was a puppy pad for spills on a black leather chair, a flat screen TV playing inspiration and a little plastic cup. Worse still, the girls at reception recognised Paul as Fisher and told him how much they liked his music. Classic.

After fertilisation, not all the embryos survived. Five dropped to three. Then two. By the end of the week, we had one viable embryo, which we decided to freeze, and one sub-optimal embryo that hadn't reached blastocyst (which is required for IVF). We were given the option of disposing of the second embryo, or implanting it. We chose the latter. It was worth a shot!

I broke the rules and did a pregnancy test before the recommended two-week wait. After peeing on the stick, I swear I saw a faint second line. The next day, my period came. Either my eyes had deceived me, or I'd experienced a chemical pregnancy, a very early miscarriage. It sucked.

Ell and I were going down the IVF stream together, in separate boats, but side by side. I felt guilty because Ell was alone, while I had Paul sitting next to me. She never for a second made me feel that way, though. She took everything in her stride. As much as we each wished things were different for the other, we were glad to have one another for support. A lot of women go through the shitstorm alone. At least Ell and I had each other to lean on.

When Ell went through her first round of IVF, she ended up with three embryos, fertilised with Chumpy's sperm. The first insemination didn't stick, but she was hopeful the second one would. I was hopeful for her, and for me.

It felt like our lives were consumed with fertility and loss and grief. Ell and I talked about those things with each other, but they almost felt like taboo topics to discuss in public. We wanted to change that. When I first floated the idea of a podcast, Ell screwed up her face and shook her head.

'Who'd want to listen to us blabber on?' she asked.

'Um, who wouldn't!?' I countered.

As usual, I eventually won her over. We mapped out a vision for a podcast all about womanhood, widowhood, grief, fertility, IVF and all the beautiful and ugly shit in between. We just had to figure out what to call it . . . Ell used to wear a t-shirt with the words 'Darling Shine' emblazoned on it, and the sentiment stuck. *Darling, Shine!* was born.

We started recording while we were both trying to fall pregnant. I was keen to do another round of IVF straight away, but I was interstate on day three of my period, so I missed my chance. Instead, we decided to do an intrauterine insemination (IUI), which is basically inseminating specially prepared sperm into the uterus during ovulation. A lot of people opt to do IUI before IVF, one reason being because it's cheaper. I went in for my trigger shot to induce ovulation, and thirty-six hours later, I was sitting in Dr Ong's chair with my legs spread. His nurse Lisa held my hand while he inserted a catheter into my cervix and released a syringe full of Paul's sperm directly in there as the eggs were coming down. Bang bang. I crossed my legs and then my fingers.

Sadly, I didn't even get a chance to do a pregnancy test because my period came early. The IUI hadn't worked. Not only did I have a low egg count, it looked like the quality was low, too. Paul's sperm had been tested, and he'd been given a gold star. He didn't have the issue. It was me.

For the first time in life, I felt a sense of resentment toward my body.

After speaking to Dr Ong, we decided to take a month off from IVF and do everything to try and improve the quality of my eggs. I began injecting myself with human growth hormones, rubbing testosterone steroid cream into my arm at night and taking melatonin. I felt like a mad scientist, researching treatments and mixing concoctions.

By the time I suited up for my next round of IVF, I was sure this was going to be the one. My eggs were going to be so healthy and juicy, and there were going to be lots of them. I willed that to be true. It had better be true – I was injecting myself with the prescribed medication six times a day! At my halfway scan, there were twelve follicles. I was pumped.

Come egg-collection day, I woke up with the number eight on my hand. Not all the follicles had grown an egg. Eight eggs were collected, but only six were mature and able to be fertilised. My odds were decreasing by the day. Overnight, I lost five eggs. When I answered the call from the clinic and they told me the news, I dropped to the floor. I was absolutely devastated. I couldn't believe that after all that, I only had one embryo.

I tried to tell myself that all it takes is one embryo. At the end of day five, the embryo was rated a Grade Five AA embryo, which is like an A+++. It is the pinnacle of embryos; you can't get any better. Finally, it felt like it was all worth it. You only need one embryo to make a baby, and I had one premium, gold-standard, high-grade embryo.

'This is going to work,' Dr Ong assured me as he prepared to inseminate the embryo into my uterus. The process was like something out of a sci-fi film. From the medical chair, I could see Dr Ong between my legs and a screen showing my uterus behind him. The lining of my uterus looked good. 'Nice and thick,' Dr Ong said.

Everything was timed to the minute. When Dr Ong pressed a button that made a 'ding dong' sound like a doorbell, the embryologist delivered my fresh embryo straight from the lab. 'Chloe Fisher, DOB 21/08/1991, one embryo,' the nurse confirmed. Dr Ong took the syringe and released the embryo inside me. I didn't feel anything – the embryo was microscopic – but I imagined it making itself at home in my uterus.

After the transfer, I wrapped myself in cotton wool to give the embryo every chance possible. Paul was in the States – he had a travel exemption for work, so he was able to leave the country – but I'd decided not to go with him. I could have joined him like I usually did – I also had a travel exemption because I ran Paul's merch and would have been working in the States – but I chose to stay on the Goldy to have the transfer.

At home, I took every precaution and then some. I became a bit pedantic about being safe and healthy. When Ell and I visited a waterfall in the Currumbin Valley, I watched as she jumped in and went swimming. I only put my feet in. I didn't want to submerge my belly in case the water temperature affected my would-be pregnancy.

I was conscious of every little flutter in my tummy. Something felt different. I sensed that I was pregnant, but I didn't dare say it out loud in case I jinxed it.

Instead, I waited the official two weeks before peeing on a stick. The test told me what I already knew: I was pregnant. The day I got the confirmation, Ell and I were set to record some bits and bobs for the podcast. I decided to tell her the good news while we were recording. 'I accidentally got a little wee on this stick,' I said, passing Ell the positive test. We both screamed with joy.

'Omg you little shit,' she said to me, giving me the biggest squeeze.

'I'm having a babyyyyy,' I squealed some more.

As it happened, we both were. Ell was seventeen weeks pregnant, but she was keeping the news on the downlow. We were chuffed to be pregnant at the same time. When I was four weeks and Ell was nineteen, we took side-by-side polaroids of our 'bumps'. Mine was non-existent – the baby was the size of a poppyseed – but I still wanted a photo. It was a pivotal moment in our lives. We were going to have babies the same year and become mothers together, just as I'd imagined when we moved to the Gold Coast.

Except, in my imaginary version of our futures, Chumpy was still here.

Your first appointment with your GP or Fertility Specialist

QUESTIONS TO ASK

- What initial tests will you recommend to assess my fertility?
- Are there any lifestyle factors that could be affecting my ability to conceive?
- How does my age impact my fertility and what does that mean for my options?

TESTING

- What blood tests or hormone tests will you run, and what will they tell us?
- Will I need an ultrasound?
- Can my partner also undergo fertility testing? If so, what tests?
- Are there any genetic tests you recommend before trying to conceive?

TREATMENT OPTIONS

- Based on my history, what fertility treatment options do you think are most suitable for me?
- What are the success rates for each option in my situation?
- Are there less invasive treatments we could try first?

- How long should we try naturally before considering assisted reproductive treatments like IUI or IVF?

LIFESTYLE AND ALTERNATIVE APPROACHES

- Are there any dietary, lifestyle or supplement recommendations that could help?
- Can stress, exercise or weight impact my fertility?
- Do you recommend acupuncture, naturopathy or other holistic approaches?

FINANCIAL AND EMOTIONAL CONSIDERATIONS

- What are the costs of fertility treatments, and is anything covered by insurance or Medicare (in Australia)?
- Do you offer payment plans or financial assistance programs?

NEXT STEPS

- What's our plan moving forward?
- How soon can we start treatment if needed?
- How often will we need follow-up appointments or testing?

Seven

PAST TENSE

I KNEW IT WASN'T A GOOD SIGN: THE FRESH, RED BLOOD IN MY underwear. It was June 2021, and I was six-and-a-half weeks pregnant. I first noticed the spotting before a flight to Sydney for a friend's birthday. I went straight to the doctor to get my bloods drawn, and the tests showed my hCG levels were normal for pregnancy. I turned from my doctor to online 'trying to conceive' (TTC) forums and support groups, searching for posts about spotting. I read stories about women who bled through their entire pregnancy. Trying to convince myself that everything was okay, I boarded my flight to Sydney, but I knew something was wrong.

When I landed in Sydney I was still concerned, so my doctor suggested going for an ultrasound. The last time I went for an ultrasound expecting to see my baby, the baby was gone. The trauma attached itself to the ultrasound, and I had developed a deep fear of having scans. I was shitting myself. Even more so when the regular ultrasound didn't show anything. The tech offered to do an internal ultrasound and kept looking for signs of life. There it was: a tiny flicker. My baby had a heartbeat.

Had.

Later that night at dinner, I felt wet. When I went to the bathroom, it looked like a massacre down there. It was as though someone had turned on a tap inside me – blood was gushing out. I didn't want to ruin my friend's dinner, so I borrowed a tampon. When I took it out later, there were massive clots. In the morning, I went to the hospital. I'd lost too much blood, I knew it wasn't right.

The doctor at the hospital refused to do another ultrasound because I'd had one the day before and it had showed a heartbeat. I tried to explain that something was wrong, but I struggled to find the words. I didn't know how to advocate for myself.

I went back to my parents' house, where I was staying, and continued to bleed. The next day, we launched *Darling, Shine!* and released the first episode of the podcast. As thousands of listeners tuned in to Ellidy and me introducing ourselves and talking about our hopes for the future, I was having an ultrasound at a women's clinic. On the screen, I saw the baby. But I didn't see the flicker.

'I'm really sorry,' the tech said. 'There's no heartbeat.'

I felt broken.

I kept bleeding. There was a haematoma – a pool of blood clots – between the wall of my uterus and the sac the baby was in.

Was.

I went through the motions: I returned to the Gold Coast, had a D&C and sent the contents for testing. I wanted to know if there were any chromosome abnormalities or explanations for the miscarriages. I was sick and tired of being told I was just 'unlucky' or that it 'mustn't have been the right time'.

I sat down with Dr Ong and requested every test under the sun. I needed to get to the bottom of what was happening. I needed answers. I needed Paul. He had been away for nine weeks, and I'd gone through the transfer and loss alone. All I wanted was to collapse into his arms.

Until I could do that, I collapsed into Ell's. I don't even know how I found the words to tell her I'd lost the baby. She'd been so excited when I surprised her with my pregnancy news, and we were both so stoked to be pregnant together. Part of me felt like I was letting her down. The future I had imagined for us was once again shattered.

Still, I was glad to have Ellidy to collapse into. I had so many good friends and my family supporting me. I was grateful to them all. But even with such a close community around me, miscarriage still felt like an inward journey. I knew no-one could go through the grief for me. I had to hold the weight myself.

The poet Leanne Laydon (@sunburntpoet) wrote me a poem.

MOONBEAMS AND RAINBOWS

Of all the gifts I dared to love
The greatest gift was you,
I tried so hard, you'll never know
The struggles I went through.
Those few short weeks and months
You were my whole world, my whole heart
And one day I will meet you,
My little moonbeam in the stars.
Till then send me a rainbow,
Promise it's going to be okay.
Watch over me little angel,
Send me a rainbow after the rain.

I always thought I'd have three kids. I knew I wanted more than one. I loved growing up with siblings and I wanted the same for my children. I'd explained as much to Dr Ong during our first appointment. That's why when my first egg retrieval resulted in a single viable embryo, we decided to freeze the embryo and do another round of IVF to collect more eggs. If I inserted the embryo right away and the pregnancy stuck, I wouldn't be able to harvest more eggs for at least ten months, likely longer. By that point, they might not be able to collect any eggs from me, my count was so low.

As much as I wanted to dive straight in and transfer my first strong embryo, I knew that if I wanted to have more than one child, I needed that embryo as a back-up. Strategically, I understood it was the right move, but that didn't make it any easier.

After my second miscarriage, I flew straight to LA to meet Paul. I needed to be with my husband, and Paul needed me as much as I needed him. The loss rocked him, too. I don't think we talk enough about the impact of miscarriages on men. Naturally, our focus goes to the mother – the one carrying the baby – but fathers feel the loss too. Not physically, but emotionally. Their pain is valid.

It wasn't until we had our first miscarriage – and then our second – that we both understood how truly heart-wrenching they are. Paul confided in me that he felt an immense amount of guilt. Before our experience with loss, one of his friends had opened up about his wife losing a pregnancy. Paul didn't know what to say. He told his friend how sorry he was, but he didn't fully grasp what they were going through or how he could help. It's something Paul still regrets to this day. I remember him calling his mate to apologise for being a shit friend.

In LA, I stepped off the IVF merry-go-round. I decided to wait for the results of all the tests I'd done with Dr Ong to come back before making any moves. In the meantime, I began a round of clomid, a medication used to treat infertility in women, which works by stimulating an increase in the amount of hormones that support ovulation. I needed to have a period before I could do more IVF anyway, so I did what I could to make that happen.

After three consecutive months on clomid, I experienced the most intense bloating of my life. I was so uncomfortable, and couldn't fit into any of my clothes.

While I was in the States, we released a podcast episode revealing Ell's baby news. She was twenty-three weeks pregnant. It had been a year since Chumpy died.

Ell was nervous to share her pregnancy with the world. She was afraid that people would think she wasn't really pregnant, that it was a delusion born out of her grief. She also worried that the morality police would criticise her for using sperm retrieved post-mortem. It should have been a happy announcement, but it was fraught with nerves.

Ell was also concerned about announcing her pregnancy so soon after I'd had a miscarriage. I tried to alleviate that worry. 'I just want to let you all know that I could not be happier for Ell,' I said in the podcast. 'We've been on this journey together from the get-go. Unfortunately, I'm not pregnant . . . but I feel like this is my pregnancy too. I'm so excited.'

Everything about the situation was bittersweet. Ell had what I wanted: a baby. And I had what she wanted: my soulmate. Because we were so close, there wasn't any envy, just empathy. We were both grateful for what we had, and all the more grateful to have each other.

Bubba Chump was due October 2021.

I thought I'd have kids before I turned thirty, but the universe had other plans. I celebrated my milestone birthday in Palm Springs, California with some girlfriends, but no baby.

As I said, I thought I'd take a break from IVF while I was in the States, but again, the universe had other plans. A new strain of Covid shut down Aussie borders in 2021, so I ended up staying overseas longer than I had anticipated. As you can probably tell by now, I'm no good at sitting on my hands and waiting, so I started researching IVF clinics in LA.

Back in Australia, the tests I'd done with Dr Ong hadn't revealed any clear answers. 'When it comes to recurrent miscarriages, it comes down to three things: age, embryo or uterine issues – or a combination of all three,' Dr Ong explained. 'You've had every investigation under the sun, and things keep coming back as normal.

'I know that's very hard to stomach. This is one of the toughest marathons. Fertility treatment often involves doing the same thing and expecting a different outcome,' he added.

That's literally the definition of insanity: doing the same thing over and over and expecting different results. No wonder I felt like I was losing my mind. Still, what choice did I have? I settled on doing more IVF. I had to do something. My dear friend Erika put together a spreadsheet for me listing the details of the top fertility doctors near me in LA.

I was starting over from the beginning. Not even the beginning, ten steps behind. I didn't have a GP in America, so I had to navigate the system on my own. I booked appointments with a couple of fertility specialists in LA and Las Vegas, but I felt like I was flying blind. It wasn't until I started seeing an acupuncturist in LA who personally recommended a doctor that I felt like I had a course of action.

At my initial appointment with my LA doctor, they were frank and straight-to-the-point. There was no fluff. I missed Dr Ong, but if this doctor was going to get me pregnant, I could handle some bluntness. They were highly regarded in their field and I respected them immensely. I was put on a new course of IVF medication and scheduled for a different program of procedures. Instead of starting with a laparoscopy, we launched straight into a full round of IVF. The doctor explained that the laparoscopy would happen during the egg retrieval.

Paul's birthday fell in the middle of my two weeks of IVF needles. He'd planned a bicycle pub crawl around Venice Beach. Even though I was mid-IVF cycle, I decided to have a couple of drinks with Paul and our friends to celebrate. I had been sober on and off for the three years we'd been trying to conceive. I'd done everything completely by the book – and that hadn't got me anywhere. After wrapping myself in so much cotton wool in my last pregnancy, and still losing the baby, I realised I couldn't stop living my life while on my quest to create life. I remember a doctor saying that having a drink here and there during the fertility journey can be a good thing, because it's relaxing and can take your mind off things. Whether I was following that advice, or whether I just really felt like a wine, I decided to toast my husband on his birthday.

We set off on our pub crawl. On the back of my electric bike, I packed an esky with my IVF needles inside. I had to have my next injection at precisely 6 pm, so I brought it along for the ride. I was riding along Venice Pier after our first few stops when I felt a little tipsy. Meanwhile, Paul and our business manager, Jenn, were past that point and having a glorious time.

On the way to the last venue on the bar hop, where we were planning to spend the rest of the evening, the front wheel of my bike clipped the back wheel of Paul's. Instead of hitting the brake, I pushed the accelerator. The force threw me onto the pier with a thud. I put my hand out to protect my face, and instead, snapped my right wrist. I knew straight away it was broken. My knee was a mess, too.

Instead of calling an ambulance (America!), a friend ordered us an Uber to the nearest hospital. In the back of the car with Paul and Jenn, we burst into laughter. We were all a bit delusional from a big day. I was no doubt running on adrenaline after my crash, and Paul and Jenn were in fine form. I was in serious pain, but for some reason I found the situation utterly hilarious. Once we started laughing, we couldn't stop. It was an uncontrollable giggle fit. The Uber driver must have thought we'd completely lost the plot. I was clearly injured – he was taking us to a hospital – but we were laughing hysterically.

Things only escalated at the hospital. Paul and Jenn had to wait in the reception area while I went into the ward to fill out all the paperwork before I could be seen. I was on my own, nursing my broken wrist, when my alarm went off. It was time to do my IVF injection. Fuck.

I tried explaining to the hospital staff member with me that I needed my husband or friend to be allowed in to give me a shot. I was right-handed, you see – I couldn't have done it myself. The staff member looked at me like I was delusional. Her eyebrows said, *What's this silly Australian doing talking about shots?*

Eventually, Jenn was allowed to come in and we went to the hospital toilets to do the injection. The needle didn't come pre-prepared, so Jenn had to mix the medication and draw the liquid into the syringe. She was doing exactly that when I noticed the blood. It was fucking everywhere. Jenn had pricked her hand on the needle and was bleeding all over the place. We couldn't stop laughing.

It was like a scene out of a Mr Bean skit, only more gory.

Eventually, I was taken to get an X-ray, which confirmed my wrist had been snapped in half. I was fitted with a very chic pink plaster cast and sent on my way.

The cotton wool was well and truly off. A week later at my egg retrieval, the doctor managed to get six eggs. In the end, the round produced two embryos. I told the doctor I didn't want to know the sex, but I did want to know if it was two of the same gender or one of each. It was the latter. A boy and a girl. I couldn't wait to tell them about the adventures of their conception.

We put our embryos on ice. My future was in a freezer.

Back home, my friends' futures were right in front of them. I'm not kidding when I say I had fifteen friends all pregnant at the same time – I counted. I didn't think I would be the person who was sensitive about pregnancy announcements and baby shower photos, but that's exactly who I became. Seeing a bump or ultrasound scan posted on Instagram felt like a knife to the throat. It was triggering and painful. Part of me was almost grateful I was stuck in America, because I don't know how I would've managed to plaster a smile on my face at baby shower after baby shower.

Still, I was crushed to be missing the birth of Ellidy's baby. When she went into labour, Ell video-called me from the maternity ward, while she was standing under a hot shower in the throes of contractions. It was late in LA and I'd had a big night. Earlier in the evening, I had made my DJ debut at a house party in Venice, where the decks were set up in the kitchen. That's how my DJ name, Kitchen Kween, was born. After the party, I headed home, stopping in at my neighbour's place for a red wine en route. I was sitting on his couch when Ell called from her birthing suite. We were in two completely different places, in every possible sense. I would have given anything to be there with her.

When I woke up the next morning, I messaged Ell's mum, Karen, straight away: *Is the baby here!?*

She was born seven minutes ago, Karen replied.

Minnie Alex Pullin was born on 25 October 2021, at 2.50 am, Australia time.

Ell asked me and Paul to be Minnie's godparents. It was an honour. I promised to look after Minnie and her mum for ever and ever.

Paul and I flew back from America to Sydney together as soon as we were allowed to. Ellidy was in Sydney too, so we met at Laura's apartment in North Narrabeen, where Minnie was fast asleep. When I finally met my goddaughter, a month after she was born, I cradled her in my arms and traced the lines of her face with my finger. She was perfect. I couldn't believe how tiny she was. Our little miracle.

'She's here,' is all I could manage to say. I couldn't speak, all I could do was stare at her. I don't know how long I sat there, looking at her, watching her chest rise and fall in her sleep.

When Minnie woke up and looked at me, I swear I saw Chumpy. She had her dad's eyes.

The bond I had with Minnie was instant, and Paul felt the same. Our love for her was intense and unconditional.

As I've said, I didn't feel any envy toward Ell over her pregnancy. I was definitely jealous of her naturally full lips and her supermodel height, but not of Minnie. I don't know if it's because we were so close or because I was so involved, but all I felt was happiness for her. And a gratefulness for being a part of her journey. Seeing Minnie wasn't triggering, it was beautiful, and hopeful.

Ell was such a natural mum. A total weapon! I knew she would be. She carried Minnie in her arms like she'd always been there.

Ell spoke to me about the pressure she felt to be both mum and dad to her baby. Chumpy's shoes were impossible to fill, but he was still so much a part of Minnie's life. He was in their dog, Rummi, in the music he made, in the home he and Ell created, and in the sky above. We started calling Chump 'Daddy in the Sky'.

A guide to holding space for grief

How to support a friend or loved one experiencing pregnancy loss, from the experts at Pink Elephants

PRACTICAL WAYS TO HELP

Let your friend feel all that she is feeling, whether it's sadness, anger or intense grief. Let her cry, and let her work through all the emotions as they come. They will most likely fluctuate day by day, and that's completely normal. Just keep on listening and supporting her by being there for her.

Cook your friend a meal or two, or arrange to have a food delivery service drop a few days' worth of food to her. Although she may not feel like eating, just the fact that she doesn't have to think about cooking will be a great relief to her.

Offer to help with other children, or to take/pick up older kids from school. Practical and specific offers of help are better than generalised, well-meaning statements like 'Let me know if I can do anything', because in most cases, your friend will feel uncomfortable or burdened to even have to think of a way you can help.

Check in every few days to see how she is doing. A simple text is enough, just to let her know that you haven't forgotten she is hurting and you haven't forgotten her loss. In your message, acknowledge that there is no need to respond, and that you just want her to know that you're thinking of her.

If you are really worried about your friend and feel her behaviour or state of mind is becoming harmful or dangerous in some way, speak to her partner or seek professional advice.

Something to bear in mind if you are pregnant (or become pregnant soon after a friend's loss) is that it may be difficult for her to be around you. Please don't be offended. Always tell your friend that you are pregnant via a text message – avoid announcing in a group setting if possible so she can have time to process on her own first. She can be happy for you and sad for her loss at the same time. If you can, let her know that you understand and respect her need for distance from you at this time, but that you're still there for her.

A woman's reaction to a miscarriage is very individual, but whatever they are feeling, they should have their feelings supported by those around them. Remember, the best way to help them is to listen, first and foremost. If, after that, you want to say something, be empathetic, loving and acknowledging of their loss.

WHAT NOT TO SAY

'It wasn't meant to be.'

Believe it or not, this really isn't helpful and it tends to shut the conversation down very quickly because your friend may feel they can't express their feelings of grief.

'You can always have another one.'

Firstly, you don't know this for sure, but more importantly, your friend wanted THAT baby. They had been dreaming of and planning for that particular baby. Another one will never be that one.

'You wouldn't have wanted a baby that had something wrong with it.'
This may be so, but it is of no comfort to her to hear that at this time. She is grieving her perfect baby, who she will never meet.

'At least you know you can get pregnant.'
Your friend is probably feeling like her body has failed her in some way and could be blaming herself for the loss, so this comment is not overly helpful and will not make her feel any better.

'Be thankful that you have your other children.'
Again, while we know this is said to focus on the positives or to cheer your friend up, all it really does is invalidate her grief. Would you say the same to someone who had lost a child?

'At least it happened early and wasn't a real baby yet.'
To your friend, from the day she saw two lines on a pregnancy test, her baby was real and very much loved. Yes, of course there is a difference between an early loss and a late-term stillbirth, but be assured your friend's baby was real and will never be forgotten.

'Miscarriage is really common . . . It happens to lots of people.'
While this may be true, in saying this, you are effectively shutting your friend down and minimising her grief. Also, please don't make comparisons to others who you know or have heard about who've had four, five, ten losses. This is her miscarriage, her loss and her grief – and for her, it's the most important loss.

'It's obviously God's will.'
Even if your friend is religious, explaining away her loss as being part of God's plan could be very hurtful to your friend. If your

friend is not religious, but you are, please leave God out of it. Just support your friend through her grief as best you can.

WHAT TO SAY

'I'm sorry for your loss.'

Simple, but full of understanding and acknowledgement.

'I'm sorry this happened.'

Again, simple yet powerful, and leaves the door open for your friend to talk and express how she is feeling.

'You must really be hurting right now.'

Recognise her pain and acknowledge it. Don't let her grief go unseen, or her baby be an elephant in the room.

'I know how much this baby meant to you.'

It means a lot to realise something precious has been lost.

'Take as long as you need to grieve.'

It may seem obvious, but sometimes it can be really helpful for your friend to feel like she has permission to be sad, particularly if her loss happened early in the pregnancy. Let her know that her grief has a place with you.

Listen and say nothing.

Sometimes even just sitting next to your friend, putting an arm around her (or not, if she's not a huggy person), can be very supportive. Tell her if she wants to talk or cry she can, or else you can sit together for as long as she needs.

Let her know if you've been through it too.

Being around people who 'get it' will be of great comfort to your friend. She will be able to express herself freely and feel safe in doing so. And most importantly, she will not feel alone.

'How is your partner coping?'

While partners may not have the physical and/or hormonal aftermath of miscarriage to deal with, they still may be grieving. It's thoughtful to ask how they are.

Eight

UNWRITTEN

It wasn't the first time I asked the universe for a sign. I was getting a manicure at home in Palm Beach and, as always, dreaming about my future child. *Come on universe, give me something,* I thought, as I perused the wall of polish options. One colour stood out to me, and I reached over to pick up the bottle. I gave it a habitual shake and turned it upside down to check the name, which was written on the bottom. 'Baby Girl.'

A sign. I was sure of it. I was going to have a baby girl . . .

I went into my fourth round of IVF holding onto an unshakeable belief: I would be a mother. I knew in my bones that I was going to have a baby, and I truly felt like I was going to carry that baby myself. Until I had a baby of my own to hold, I had to hold onto that belief.

I started to live by the mantra 'whatever will be, will be'. I told myself that my story was already written. If my fourth round of IVF was going to be successful, it would be. If it was going to be unsuccessful, it would be. There was nothing I could do to change the story already set in stone.

I tried to surrender to the universe. Some days that was easier than others.

On 1 February 2022, when I had an embryo from my fourth round of IVF transferred, I was given a black-and-white photo of the embryo. I couldn't stop looking at it. All my hopes and dreams in one tiny image.

At some point, the embryo in the photo – the embryo inside me – split in two. I was carrying identical twin boys. The universe had told me about a baby girl, not twin boys, but I wasn't going to argue. I was pregnant, that was all I cared about. I just had to stay that way.

I held onto my unshakable belief, I held onto the black-and-white photo of my embryo, and I held onto hope.

But no matter how tightly I held, I couldn't save my babies. Our story was already written.

As you already know, I lost the twins – first one, and then the second. It was soul-crushing. After our makeshift ceremony on the beach with the white roses, I felt an immense need to get away.

I was so fucking over it. My hands were sore from clinging onto hope. I gave up and let go. I booked a flight to the States, where Paul was playing Miami Music Week, and landed in the arms of a group of strangers. Brett and his girlfriend, Tallara, had organised for us to spend the week on their friends' superyacht, but I arrived before Brett and Paul, so I boarded the boat on my own. I was welcomed by the most divine women, who I hadn't met before. In the arms of those strangers, I completely fell apart. 'I had a miscarriage two weeks ago,' I shared between tears. 'I lost twins.'

For the rest of the week, the women nurtured and cared for me. One of them practised reiki and gave me a healing session. Another led a full moon ceremony on the top deck. They all gave me space to cry, and talk, and be silent. It was exactly what I needed in the moment, and those women are still my very good friends to this day.

I took a month off social media and focused on being present and spending time with Paul. It was incredible to see him performing to sold-out crowds, getting recognised on the street, and generally being in his element. Things really started to take off for Paul after 'Losing It', but just as he was picking up momentum, the world shut down. The entire music industry took a huge hit during the pandemic. Without live gigs, artists, venues, roadies, managers, band members, light technicians and sound engineers all suffered. It felt cruel that

Paul had worked so hard for so many years to get to where he was, only for the whole industry to come to a standstill.

We were lucky to be able to ride out the lockdowns and come out the other side; plenty of other artists weren't as fortunate. Needless to say, I was stoked to be going to gigs again and seeing the music industry clawing its way back.

After a month on the road, I returned to Australia for a stint – and another round of IVF – before we headed to Ibiza for Paul's 2022 residency and a score of Euro summer shows. Let's be honest: I came home for Minnie. I couldn't get enough of her. Paul and I would take her out to the shops or on walks to give Ell a rest. We doted on Minnie like she was our own. And she was – she was our goddaughter. Besides, Minnie was easy to dote on. She was such a good baby. She could – and would – sleep anywhere, and she was always smiley and happy to see you.

I felt like I'd missed out on so much of Minnie while I was away in the States, and I didn't want to miss any more. So, we invited Ell and Minnie to join us in Ibiza.

I'll never forget the moment they arrived in Spain. It was after midnight when Ell landed, after more than twenty-four hours of travelling from Australia. She was carrying Minnie, who was then ten months old, her nappy bag, handbag and a stroller. She must have been completely and utterly exhausted. I didn't realise at the time just how big it was for her to travel to the other side of the world with a little baby on her own.

And yet, Ell did it with such grace. Even when her luggage was lost in transit!

After touching down in Ibiza, we took Ell and Minnie home to our villa, where we had a babysitter ready to go. Paul's set was on at 3 am, and Ell was keen to go. I genuinely don't know how she mustered the energy. She had no clothes to wear, so Paul took pity on her and loaned her one of his precious Balenciaga shirts. She looked fantastic in it. She's the definition of that *Mean Girls* meme, 'I'm not a regular mom, I'm a cool mom.' I was in awe of her.

Doing Ibiza with a baby was a totally different experience. My favourite memories from our 2022 Euro summer include feeding Minnie spaghetti in the shower because she was so messy; watching her gnaw on steak at restaurants; seeing her fall in love with the cat at our villa; swimming with her in the Mediterranean Sea; and taking her to her first festivals.

It was Minnie's appearance at the Family Piknik Festival in France that went viral. Ell was standing next to me side-stage with Minnie in a carrier on her chest, wearing an adorable pair of pink headphones to protect her ears. Paul was flicking his wrist to the beat, pumping up the crowd and playing peek-a-boo with Minnie. She was completely mesmerised, and had the most enormous smile on her face. We shared a video of the moment online and it went totally nuts. Minnie's first rave was viewed millions and millions of times, and she became an icon in the scene. People started bringing giant cut-outs of her face to gigs, making their own merch with 'Minnie Moo' written in caps, and holding signs that said 'Where's Minnie?'

Paul reckons people would get pissed off at him when Minnie wasn't at his show. 'It's 1 am, she's in bed, mate. She's a baby,' he'd explain.

That Euro summer was the first time Paul had a dedicated plane to get him to all of his gigs. Flying on a private jet was a surreal experience for us, but Minnie didn't know any different. 'Don't get used to this life, doll, we're flying economy home,' Ell joked to her.

While Paul was busy doing shows, we had a girls' weekend in Paris. We went to the Formula 1 Dutch Grand Prix in Amsterdam (where Minnie met Daniel Ricciardo), and dined at the five-star Six Senses Resort back in Spain (where Minnie ate kingfish carpaccio). Our very best day, though, was spent on a boat off Es Vedrà island, west of Ibiza. We were there with the fam (Ell and Minnie) and our mates Karina, Laura and Jake. We swam in the sea, watched the sunset and danced into the night. In between it all, we cuddled Minnie. It was one of those never-forget, picture-perfect afternoons.

This might sound woo-woo, but the area had such a spiritual and magical feeling. The small rocky island is 400 metres tall and uninhabited by humans. In ancient mythology, it is said to be home to the Phoenician goddess Tanit, who is worshipped as the patron goddess of fertility.

I didn't plan that. But even in the middle of the Mediterranean Sea, far away from my embryos in Australia, fertility was still at the front of my mind. I was having the most incredible experiences with the people I loved the most, and still, my mind was consumed with the thought of having a baby. I couldn't escape it.

On Instagram, my life looked like one big party – and in so many ways it was. But the yacht shots on the Mediterranean Sea didn't show the invisible weight I was carrying everywhere I went. Unless someone was following my personal journey on *Darling, Shine!*, they wouldn't have had a clue what I was going through. I spoke about the reality on the podcast, but I didn't share my day-to-day struggles. No-one saw the late-night tears over my lost babies. No-one saw my deep longing.

No-one except for Paul. He had the same longing, but it was different for him. It wasn't his body that was letting us down. Our inability to have a baby was tough on our relationship. Paul struggled being away so much for work and not being by my side for every appointment. He felt helpless. When something terrible happened, he would cancel shows and fly straight home, but he couldn't always be there for the moments in between, which some days were just as hard.

Paul always tried to make things better for me. He went above and beyond to fill the baby-shaped hole in our lives. When I was having a down day, he would do his best to distract me. 'Come on, let's go do something fun. Let's go out for dinner, or go and grab an ice-cream,' he would say. It was lovely of him, but more often than not, I just didn't have the energy to go out and pretend to be happy. I was physically and emotionally exhausted.

My entire existence revolved around my hormonal cycle. I tracked my ovulation every day. I filled my schedule with fertility appointments. I spent every waking hour doing research, reading books and listening to podcasts. I became quite obsessive.

I'm lucky that my relationship with Paul is so strong, because I know a lot of relationships have derailed on the IVF roller-coaster.

Paul could see the toll it was taking on me. 'I think we should take a break. Let's give your body a breather,' he said.

But I was adamant. 'I'm not stopping until I have a baby.'

Paul was only trying to help, but I didn't see it that way. I was frustrated that he would even suggest having a break. I felt like I didn't have time to waste. I needed to knuckle down and get shit done. I was fully committed to the cause.

I returned to Australia in the last week of October 2022, and my period arrived on the 31st. It was like a sign. I could start doing a round of IVF straight away. I began doing the injections two days later and braced myself for the bruised tummy that would come. I realised my stomach had been covered in bruises for the better part of two years. Surely it was all going to pay off!

After ten days of needles, my trigger shot – the hormone injection I needed to do exactly thirty-six hours before the egg retrieval – was timed for 6.30 pm on 12 November. As fate would have it, Paul was playing a gig in Sydney that night. His set time was 7.30 pm. I was in the green room backstage at the Domain, hanging out with all my friends and Paul's crew and keeping an eye on the time. I told my mates about the injection I was about to do and they cheered me on. Everyone kissed my belly and wished me good luck.

Just as I was about to jab myself in the tummy, Matt and Jack from the comedy duo The Inspired Unemployed walked into the room. 'What are you doing?' they asked, slightly alarmed at the needle I had pressed against my bare stomach.

'Oh, I'm doing IVF and this is my trigger shot,' I explained.

Their faces were blank. Still, they tried to be encouraging and started chanting, 'IBS! IBS! IBS!'

Close, but not quite.

I swear all the blokes in the room thought I was injecting Paul's sperm into my stomach. It was pretty hilarious. I focused on soaking up all the good energy in the room and channelling it into my womb.

Paul played a killer gig to a sold-out Domain. He had shows in Perth and Brisbane the following week, but I wasn't able to join him. I had to be on the Gold Coast for my egg retrieval.

Once again, I was going through the procedure alone. My friend Erika drove me to the clinic and held my hand.

In the five days that followed, six eggs became four eggs, which resulted in two embryos. We had those embryos genetically tested, and one came back normal, while the other one was 'mosaic', meaning it had both normal and abnormal cells. Mosaic embryos can develop into healthy babies; however, they carry a higher chance of miscarriage. That was the last thing I needed. We froze the two embryos and used our already frozen embryo from the first round of IVF in the transfer.

It was my first time having a frozen embryo transferred, and it was my first embryo to have been collected. I decided in my mind that this was going to be the one. My first embryo was going to be my first earthside baby. I prayed for it to be so.

The week following my transfer, Paul and I headed to Sydney together. He was nominated for Artist of the Year at the *GQ* Men of the Year Awards. It was a big night in the world of magazine publishing. Actor Russell Crowe, sportsman Dylan Alcott and Prime Minister Anthony Albanese were on the guest list. There was a plush red carpet, and an ice luge overflowing with caviar and Belvedere Vodka. I had my hair and make-up done and was wearing the most glorious KYHA Studios gown.

I squealed with joy when Paul won the award – Artist of the Year! – and again when he mentioned me in his acceptance speech. 'I want to thank my lovely wife,' he said. 'Thank you for letting me be me, because I know I can be a pest, most of the time. I just want to thank you. Every time we go to a club or have a party, you're always there by my side and they're the greatest moments I could have. Thank you, babe, I love you.'

Everyone around me was getting loose and enjoying the free drinks, but I wasn't partaking. I did a pregnancy test before the big night, but it came back negative. I hoped it was just too early to tell and was on my best behaviour, just in case.

My period came three days later. Part of me kicked myself for not letting my hair down at the party. How many moments had I wasted, holding back, hoping for a pregnancy that didn't eventuate? I'd lost count.

Steps forward – healing after loss

- Society often downplays pregnancy loss, but your grief is real. Acknowledge your feelings and give yourself permission to mourn.
- Say no and ask for space when you need it to allow yourself to heal.
- Set boundaries. A simple response – 'I appreciate your support, but I need space right now' – can be helpful when you're in the thick of grief.
- Your body might still feel pregnant after loss. Be gentle with yourself. Eat nourishing foods and drinks and rest when needed.
- Connect with people who understand – whether through a support group, a therapist, or a close friend.
- Honour your baby in a way that feels right for you. Some ideas that I have used . . .
    - Name your baby.
    - Plant a tree or garden.
    - Sponsor a star.
    - Light a candle.
    - Write them a letter.
    - Let flowers drift out to sea.

Question prompts for hopeful mothers and fathers

In 2021, Paul and I sat down to answer these questions together as we navigated our fertility journey. The answers were revealing, and helped us reflect and look forward. We both answered that we were excited to travel the world together with our baby. Paul said he was most afraid of the baby not thinking their dad was cool (he was joking), and I said I was afraid of not becoming pregnant, of having another miscarriage and of the toll it might take on our relationship.

'The process feels REAL and tough at times, but when it happens, it's going to be magic,' Paul wrote.

What does becoming a mother/father mean to me?
What am I looking forward to?
What am I not looking forward to?
My fears are . . .
The process feels . . .

Nine

NUMB

At this point, I need to break the fourth wall and speak directly to you. Are you exhausted reading this story? Because I'm exhausted telling it. By the end of 2022, I felt like I was reliving Groundhog Day, day after day, month after month, cycle after cycle. It was a never-ending roller-coaster of hope followed by despair. Up and down, up and down.

If it sounds tiring, that's because it is. This is the reality of infertility. It fucking sucks.

I became numb to the disappointment. 'Righto, let's go again,' I said when my *fifth* embryo transfer didn't work. And so, we did.

I had previously done a test to see if I had Natural Killer (NK) cells and my levels came back normal. But because of my recurrent miscarriages and unsuccessful rounds of IVF, I was treated for them anyway. From day one of my period in December 2022, I started taking a low dose of aspirin, which is commonly used to prevent eclampsia. Come day three, I began taking prednisolone, a steroid which reduces inflammation and is given to women who experience recurrent miscarriage. On top of that, I was doing Clexane injections to stop blood clots forming in the embryo and placenta. It was a full concoction.

My egg retrieval in mid-December only collected four eggs. It was a hard pill to swallow. I knew the average number of eggs collected during IVF was between eight and fifteen. I'd been in the clinic when women had twenty and thirty collected. Four felt pitiful.

The numbness had worn off and I felt the full weight of the disappointment. It was fucking heavy.

When the clinic rang me later that night, they gently told me that only one of the eggs was mature. The next morning, they rang to say the single mature egg hadn't survived the night. I'd done a full round of IVF – my eighth – and I had nothing to show for it. Not an egg. Not an embryo. And not a baby. I didn't know it then, but my eighth round of IVF would be my last.

The sorrow I felt was similar to the sadness of having a miscarriage. It felt like a loss. A waste of a month. A punch to the gut.

I went ahead and transferred the frozen embryo from the month before (the one that came back normal on the genetic test). It was late December and the silly season was in full swing. Everyone was throwing Christmas parties, drinking champagne and sliding into holiday mode. I wasn't. I didn't feel like celebrating.

I started bleeding on Boxing Day. *Another round bites the dust,* I thought to myself. Fucking hell. I stopped taking the progesterone capsules I'd been prescribed for the pregnancy.

The next day I went to the beach with Ell and Minnie. The sky was moody, and I felt the same. I swam out into the ocean alone and looked up at the clouds. I spoke to Chumpy. 'Come on Chump, can you pull a few strings up there and help us out?' I said to him.

I was standing under the beach shower when my phone rang. I recognised the number as my IVF clinic. When I answered, I thought I heard a note of happiness in the clinician's voice as she asked me to confirm my name and date of birth. 'So, your blood tests have come back and you're pregnant,' the woman said. 'It's positive.'

I nearly fell backward. It caught me completely off guard. Doing IVF takes all the surprise out of pregnancy, so it was a shock to be shocked. I screamed out to Ell, who was in the car park buckling Minnie into her car seat. She jumped up and down. At home, I peed on a stick and the two lines were clear. It was positive. I was pregnant.

I was so, so happy to be pregnant – for the fourth time – but I couldn't let myself feel the happiness. After three miscarriages, all I could feel was nerves and anxiety.

Miscarriage robbed me of my innocence. I would never get to experience the joy of pregnancy again. Miscarriage wouldn't let me. It stole the joy and replaced it with fear.

Worst of all, I had every reason to be afraid.

I didn't know if the bleeding I'd thought was my period was spotting of old blood, or the kind of spotting that can happen in early pregnancy. I just hoped it wasn't a bad sign. Worryingly, my hCG levels were low, and my progesterone was too. I had stopped taking my progesterone capsules when I thought my period had started, so I missed a day's worth of the hormones. The clinic advised me to take one every two hours to boost my levels.

Because of the low levels and the bleeding, I didn't let myself get excited about the positive pregnancy test.

At my next scan, three days later, my levels were slowly rising. My hCG levels were supposed to double every day, and they weren't quite doing that, but they were very close. I was booked in for an ultrasound to check if I was having an ectopic pregnancy. I was only around six weeks, so it was early for an ultrasound, but we wanted to know what was going on. The numbers weren't adding up the way we wanted them to.

Paul and I were booked in to see the same ultrasound technician we had when we lost our twins. The poor thing. She couldn't see anything in my uterus. She tried so hard to spot something. She even called in the gynaecologist on duty to re-do the scan and double check. There was nothing in my tubes, so it wasn't an ectopic pregnancy. As the ultrasound tech zoomed in on my uterus, she said she thought she could see an adhesion, but she couldn't be sure. The possibility stuck with me.

We walked out of the ultrasound clinic in the same state of uncertainty as when we'd walked in. I didn't know if it was just too early, and the baby was too small, for the scan to show anything, or if the baby wasn't there. Either way, we didn't have any answers.

My bloods still said I was pregnant, so I acted accordingly. When we had a big Hard Fizz event, I poured soda water into an empty can, so people didn't realise I wasn't drinking and ask me about it. Someone caught me swapping out the alcohol and she raised her eyebrows and looked at my tummy, wordlessly asking if I was pregnant. The answer was too complicated to explain.

Because I was so open about our fertility journey on *Darling, Shine!* and my social media, people were invested in what was happening. I understand that, and I appreciate all the care and support I've been shown, but it can be hard going through something so vulnerable with an audience. I hated the pressure of people watching to see if I was drinking or not, or if I went to one of Paul's gigs or not, or if I was bloated or not.

I became more careful about how much I shared. Not just because of the added pressure I was feeling, but because I didn't want to talk about it. And mostly, because I genuinely didn't know what was happening.

I decided not to tell people that I was pregnant because things were so touch and go. Then my Pop had a heart attack. He had been raced to the hospital in Sydney and resuscitated in the ambulance on the way there. The doctors said he wouldn't survive the night. My mum video-called me from the hospital so I could say goodbye while he was still conscious. I had to tell him I was pregnant. I wanted him to tell Grandma and Chumpy.

'Poppa, we're pregnant,' I said. I felt proud saying those words out loud.

'That's the best news ever,' Poppa said.

The next day, the hospital turned off the adrenaline that was keeping Pop alive. Somehow, he stayed alive. His body should have shut down, but it didn't. He kept fighting. I wanted to give him something to fight for, I wanted to give him his first great-grandchild.

But even though I'd said it out loud, the pregnancy still didn't feel real.

I had a weekend away booked in Byron Bay, and I ummed and ahhed about going because we were in such a state of unknown with the pregnancy. I decided to push ahead. Paul had an overseas gig, so I went on my own. As soon as I checked into the hotel, the IVF clinic called. 'Your levels seem to have plateaued.'

As if on cue, I started to bleed heavily. I called my friends Tash and Bianca, who were in Byron too, and they rushed to my side. We had planned to meet for dinner, where I was going to tell them I was pregnant. Instead, we sat in the hotel room and cried. Tash had experienced a miscarriage weeks earlier, so we cried for ourselves and each other.

The next day, I went to a pathology clinic in Byron to have more blood taken. The results were sent to Dr Ong, who told me my levels were rising again. 'You have to continue to be pregnant until you're not pregnant,' Dr Ong said. 'If your levels are rising, there's still something growing in there.'

Deep down, I think the doctor knew the numbers weren't viable – even though they were rising, they weren't rising the way they should be – but he couldn't say so. It was like I had to keep telling myself I was pregnant until I actively miscarried.

I wanted to pull my hair out. One day my levels said I was pregnant, the next they didn't. One day I was bleeding, the next I wasn't. It was such a headfuck.

By week nine, the bleeding had stopped, and I was getting my levels tested every three days. I was due to fly to Bali the following week, when Dr Ong called. 'Have you been bleeding?' he asked.

'No, I haven't had any bleeding,' I said.

He paused.

'I'm so sorry, but your levels have completely dropped,' Dr Ong said. 'You're having your fourth miscarriage. If you're not bleeding already, you will be,' he continued.

It was the moment we had all been waiting for. Even though I'd known it was coming, the hit still hurt. I asked Dr Ong to book me in for a D&C the next day, but he told me I would have to wait until I started bleeding. It felt cruel. We knew the baby was gone, but I wasn't able to have it removed. I couldn't bear the thought of the lost baby inside me.

On 25 January 2023, I wrote in my journal . . .

Miscarriage #4 WTF

The past four weeks have been nothing short of torture. Four weeks of the highs and the lows, the hopes and the dashed dreams. I would have been eight weeks pregnant today, but instead I am grieving the loss of my fifth baby. My HCG levels crept up and up until yesterday, when they dropped from 2400 to 1200. Just gutted. For some reason I had so much hope that this was the one: an A Grade embryo, genetically tested and healthy. What is going on!? I just don't get it. Fuck.

I had the D&C as soon as I could, then I boarded a flight to Bali. Back to where it all began.

Hotel Komune is located on a volcanic beach on the east coast of Bali. The sand is black, the waves are crisp, and the sun is powerful. I've always found Bali to be an incredibly healing place, but I especially feel that way about Komune. We were staying in a villa there in February 2023 with Ellidy and Minnie. That's where we found out my pop had passed away after his heart attack two weeks earlier.

I hadn't told him I'd lost the baby. He died thinking I was pregnant. I don't know if that's better or worse, but I'm glad he wasn't worried or upset for me when he left us.

The morning I found out about my pop, I had booked in for a water healing ceremony in the rainforest mountains of Ubud. When I arrived, the healer immediately asked about my grandparents, and told me I had a woman spirit who followed me down the track to the waterfall. It gave me goosebumps. I've always felt my grandma's spirit in Bali, the place where she died, and the healer confirmed my feeling.

I decided not to fly back to Australia for Poppa's funeral. Instead, we held a Balinese ceremony for him, just as we had done with Grandma. We went down to the black-sand beach with a local priest and farewelled my poppa. I said goodbye in my own way. It felt right. Of course, it was hard not being with my family after Poppa's passing, but I still tried to honour and remember him.

I know my brother was disappointed that I didn't come back for Poppa's funeral. That's understandable. He was grieving in his own way – with the extended family – and I was too. Cooper apologised to me later for making me feel guilty about my decision.

It might have been selfish of me, but after what I'd been through in the previous few weeks and months, I didn't want to put my body through another long-haul flight if I could help it. I knew Poppa would understand, and I made peace with my choice.

I felt that I needed to be in Bali at that very moment in time to heal and make sense of the loss of our fourth pregnancy and fifth baby. In Ellidy's hotel room overlooking Uluwatu Beach, we recorded a *Darling, Shine!* episode.

'I've got three embryos in Australia and two in the States, so I'm hoping that within those five, one of them will work. And at this point, if I could have one baby, I would be so grateful for that,' I said, mentioning that we were also looking into surrogacy as an option. 'I'm going to the States, and I'm going to my doctor in LA. I want them to start from scratch [with tests and examinations]. I need a fresh pair of eyes.

'I really do believe there is something going on with my uterus, because I'm thirty-one years old, using genetically tested embryos, and losing them before nine weeks every time,' I continued.

Something was wrong, and I was going to find out what it was. I wasn't going to put up with being told I was just unlucky, or that some things were unexplainable. I wanted an explanation. I needed one.

How to advocate for yourself in the medical system

The medical system can be overwhelming, frustrating and, at times, completely disheartening. But if there's one thing I've learned through my own journey, it's this: you have to be your own biggest advocate. No-one will fight for your health the way you will. Doctors are experts, but they don't live in your body – you do. If something doesn't feel right, speak up. If you feel dismissed, push harder. If you don't understand something, ask again.

Here's how I took care of myself during my fertility journey.

TRUST YOUR GUT – IT'S ALWAYS RIGHT

If something feels off, it probably is. Don't let anyone, no matter how qualified they are, brush aside your concerns. You deserve to be heard, respected and taken seriously. Keep pushing until you get the answers you need.

THIS IS THE BIGGEST POINT, IN MY EYES – KNOWLEDGE IS POWER

Understanding your body and your health is one of the most powerful things you can do! Research your symptoms (to an extent . . . remember, Google isn't gospel!). Learn about possible conditions, and familiarise yourself with treatment options. You don't have to be a doctor, but knowing the basics will give you confidence in conversations with them.

ASK ALL THE QUESTIONS (YES, *ALL* OF THEM!)

Never worry that you're being annoying – this is your health we're talking about! Some key questions to ask your doctor:

- What exactly does this diagnosis mean?
- What are all the treatment options available to me?
- What are the risks and benefits of this procedure/medication?

You can refer to 'Your first appointment with your GP or Fertility Specialist' on page 90 for more examples too.

And if something still doesn't sit right? Get a second opinion. Or a third. Keep asking until you feel confident.

KEEP A PAPER TRAIL

Medical appointments can be a blur, especially when you're processing heavy information. Write everything down. In your phone notes, keep track of:

- symptoms (dates, times, severity, triggers – take photos and save them in a folder)
- medications (what's working, what's not, side effects)
- test results and reports (save in an easily accessible folder on your desktop or phone)
- top-line information from conversations with your doctors (including who said what and when).

BRING BACKUP – A SUPPORT PERSON IS EVERYTHING

Bring a partner, friend or family member. They can take notes, ask questions, and be an extra voice when you're feeling overwhelmed. You don't have to do this alone. There are so many people out there who have walked this road and *get it!* Look for online communities, local support groups or advocacy organisations.

IF YOU NEED MORE TESTS, PUSH FOR THEM

If you're being told 'It's probably fine' but you don't feel fine, insist on more testing, or get a second opinion. Ask for scans, bloodwork or a specialist referral.

FOLLOW UP IN WRITING (BECAUSE EMAILS GET ATTENTION!)

If you're struggling to get answers, send an email. A written communication trail creates a dated record, and often gets better results than endless phone calls. It also ensures your concerns aren't forgotten or misinterpreted.

Comprehensive testing

When it comes to recurrent pregnancy loss, tests can be done on the following:

- male and female karyotype
- AMH, LH, FSH, oestradiol
- TSH prolactin, testosterone
- full blood count
- cardiolipin antibodies, lupus anticoagulant
- Protein C, Protein S, antithrombin III
- APCR
- Factor V Leiden
- prothrombin gene mutation
- MTHFR mutation
- fasting glucose, insulin, homocysteine
- thyroid antibodies
- peripheral blood activated natural killer cells
- uterine natural killer cells and other endometrial pathology
- pelvic ultrasound scan
- hysteroscopy (and sometimes laparoscopy)
- semen analysis and sperm DNA fragmentation.

Ten

ANSWERS

After all the bad phone calls I'd had – 'I'm sorry, your transfer was unsuccessful', 'I'm sorry, you've lost the baby', 'I'm sorry, Poppa has died' – one call finally broke me.

Reluctantly, after my fourth miscarriage, I made an appointment with a surrogacy counsellor at the start of 2023. On the call, I said I was ready to explore surrogacy as an avenue. I told the counsellor about my journey so far, the tests, the transfers, the losses. I explained that I didn't think I could continue down the path I was on. I couldn't handle another miscarriage – I knew it would push me over the edge, and I didn't know if I would be able to crawl back up. I was sure if I lost another baby, I would also lose myself.

The counsellor listened, and then he talked me through the surrogacy process. It was a lot to take in.

When I hung up the phone, I burst into tears. For the first time, I seriously considered that I might not be able to carry my own baby. I'd been holding onto the string of my unflinching belief for so long. When I let it go, I felt empty.

I realised I wanted to be pregnant just as much as I wanted to have a baby. I wanted the whole experience – the belly, the birth, the breastfeeding. The call with the surrogacy counsellor made me doubt that would ever happen. It felt like admitting defeat.

But I wasn't going down without a fight.

When I arrived in LA in March 2023, I walked straight into an appointment with my LA fertility doctor and demanded answers. I explained that I wasn't going through another round of IVF or an embryo transfer until I got to the bottom of why I was losing my pregnancies. I told them I wanted them to take a serious look at my uterus, because I thought we could find answers there.

The doctor did as I asked. They performed a laparoscopy and found scar tissue – so much scar tissue, too much scar tissue – in my uterus. By that point, I'd had four D&Cs and the resultant scarring was significant. The doctor came up with a hypothesis. They suggested I was losing my babies before nine weeks because they could grow to a certain point before the scar tissue stopped the blood flow to the embryo and prevented it from growing further.

'This condition is called Asherman's syndrome,' the doctor explained. 'It's when scar tissue builds up inside your uterus and reduces the space in there – like the walls of a room getting thicker, making the space inside smaller.'

'I'm not going to do another transfer until you get this sorted, because you don't have enough embryos to be wasting them,' they told me. 'Once we know the soil in there is fresh, we will try again.'

I was pissed. Not necessarily at the doctor, but at the situation. I had been actively trying to fall pregnant for three years, had done eight rounds of IVF and suffered four devastating losses. If the scar tissue was the reason behind my miscarriages, why hadn't it been picked up sooner? I had done every test under the sun. I had taken every medication recommended. I had been poked and prodded and scanned by countless doctors. Why was I only now hearing of Asherman's syndrome?

There isn't a lot of research into the prevalence of Asherman's, but it is estimated that only one to five people in every 10,000 experience it. It looked like I was one of them.

I was told I needed surgery. The doctor said Dr Camran Nezhat was the best in the business, and that he specialised in Asherman's syndrome surgery. They insisted that he was the surgeon I had to have. Dr Nezhat was based in San Francisco.

So not only would I have to have – and pay for – an invasive surgery, I would also have to travel to another city to get it done. My doctor refused to do any more IVF or transfers with me until I had the surgery done. According to them, Dr Nezhat was my last shot. But they assured me I was in good hands.

I contacted Dr Kee Ong to talk through what I had been told. He disagreed with the Asherman's diagnosis and warned me about getting taken for a ride.

I was conflicted, but I felt like I didn't have a choice – I had to have the surgery. At a hefty, *hefty* cost. I didn't have health insurance in America, so I had to cover the full cost of the surgery. I justified the price by telling myself it was an investment into our future. I knew it was an investment we could only afford to make once.

In San Francisco, Dr Nezhat greeted me with a dazzling smile. He told me all the things I wanted to hear. 'Don't worry, once I'm done with you, you're going to have a baby,' he assured me.

I travelled to San Fran with my friend Tallara because Paul had gigs he couldn't miss. We checked into our hotel room, and I began to prep for my surgery with an enema. Poor Tallara.

Because I'd had so many surgeries in the last few years, I was blasé about this one. I joked that I went under anaesthetic just to get a decent rest. I actually loved the feeling of being put under and rousing from a deep sleep.

I should have known from the enema that it was going to be more full-on than the other procedures I'd had. The surgery went for over two hours, which was significantly longer than the ten minutes a D&C took. It involved Dr Nezhat cutting and removing the scar tissue in my uterus using instruments inserted through the cervix, then inflating a medical balloon to keep the uterine cavity open and prevent re-adhesion.

I knew as soon as I woke up from the operation that I had underestimated how serious it was. I felt like I had been hit by a truck. No, not a truck, a road train. I had a catheter inserted and a drainage bag. I also had an intrauterine device (IUD) implanted to release estrogen to help with healing. I only knew IUDs to be birth control – the complete opposite of what I wanted – so it felt counterintuitive to have one inside me.

It was awkward and painful to walk. Tallara helped me into our Uber, and I proceeded to spew the whole way back to our hotel. Again, poor Tallara (and the poor Uber driver).

I had never felt this bad before, and I was scared. I immediately called my mum. 'I need you,' I said, through tears. 'I need you to come and look after me, please. Can you get on the next flight to America?'

And that's exactly what she did. My mum dropped everything and flew across the world to take care of me. She was literally my guardian angel. I was so relieved when she arrived. I was a thirty-one-year-old grown woman with a husband and a mortgage, and I had never needed my mum more.

For five days, I sat in my hotel bed binge-watching *Love Island*, until I got clearance to fly. Tallara brought me room service and helped me to the bathroom.

When he gave me the green light to travel, Dr Nezhat told me how bad my Asherman's syndrome had been. 'This was a severe case,' he said, explaining that my scar tissue was especially thick because of my history of endometriosis, D&Cs and hysteroscopies. 'The adhesions weren't just in your uterus, but also inside your abdomen. Everything was very, very scarred.'

Several weeks later, back in LA with Paul, we went to see the fertility doctor to have the IUD removed. I was still tender and felt vulnerable sitting in the chair. I was glad to have Paul there holding my hand.

As the doctor was looking inside me, they said something that sent my heart racing. 'You'll need to have the surgery again to make sure it worked,' they told me.

'Um, what?' I replied. 'I'm not having that surgery again. That's not an option.'

I was adamant, but they were too.

If I was told at the beginning that I'd need to have the surgery twice, I doubt I would have gone through with it. The cost, pain and recovery time were hectic. I wasn't in a position to go to San Fran and endure that whole ordeal again. It wasn't going to happen.

We were at loggerheads. I wasn't backing down. 'I have a right as a patient to tell you what I want to do. I know this isn't what you want me to do, but I am not having the surgery again,' I said.

The doctor sighed. 'Well, let me try and do a sonohysterogram on you in the chair,' they relented. The procedure involved inserting dye inside me and using an ultrasound to see if there was any scar tissue remaining.

'Oh look, it's still there,' they said, showing me the scan.

'You've got to be kidding me,' I replied.

'There's still scarring.'

'Well, I'm not having the surgery again. We need to talk about other options.'

'Alright, let me get some saline and see if I can use it to break away some of the scar tissue,' the doctor offered.

I wasn't given any pain relief before they proceeded to squirt the saline inside me, scraping the sides of my uterus. The pain was unbearable. I was shaking and writhing in the chair. Paul was almost in tears beside me, watching the agony I was in.

'Do you need to leave the room?' the doctor asked him.

'No, I'm just fucking losing it watching my wife die in this chair,' he said.

It was brutal. When the doctor said they couldn't really do what they wanted, I told them I needed them to stop. I couldn't take a second more.

The doctor sat me up in the chair and told me I only had two options: have the surgery again, or try surrogacy. 'Don't try and fall pregnant again, because if you do, you will miscarry,' they said. Then they left the room.

I stood and went to clean myself up, but when I looked at the floor, I froze. During the procedure, I'd felt liquid coming out of me and assumed it was the saline. It wasn't. It was blood. There was blood everywhere. It was a literal blood bath. I was too shocked to cry. Paul and I just looked at each other with wide eyes. 'What the fuck just happened?'

We walked out of that doctor's clinic that day and never went back.

A spotlight on Asherman's syndrome

'Asherman's syndrome is a condition where scar tissue is present in the uterus,' explains Dr Nezhat. 'It can occur as a result of several things: a miscarriage followed by an infection, a D&C, postpartum bleeding after a birth leading to infection, endometriosis and associated surgeries.'

The exact number of people with Asherman's syndrome is unknown, but there is a higher prevalence in people who are struggling with infertility. 'Unfortunately, Asherman's is not too uncommon among patients who have had miscarriages and the above-mentioned issues,' admits Dr Nezhat.

Some people with Asherman's syndrome don't experience symptoms. Others notice lighter periods or no periods at all. Infertility and miscarriage are, sadly, the most significant symptoms. To diagnose Asherman's, further investigations are needed. 'In cases where the patient is younger, you do a sonohysterogram, an ultrasound, or a hysteroscopy to look inside the uterus,' says Dr Nezhat.

At present, the recommended treatment for Asherman's is surgery. 'When there is Asherman's – and also when there is endometriosis, in my opinion – the best treatment is surgery. We can go in and analyse all the adhesions in the uterus and fix it up by freeing the scar tissue. We then put a balloon in the uterus, and sometimes an IUD as well, to decrease the risk of collapsing the uterus and give hormonal therapy to build the endometrium again,' adds Dr Nezhat.

It is common for doctors to recommend a 'second look' after the first surgery, especially in severe cases.

It is also common, however, for people to fall pregnant after the surgery. 'I've been very lucky to work with many patients who get pregnant naturally after the surgery. It is very common,' says Dr Nezhat. 'I feel very lucky [to do this work]. I remember a patient from a long time ago who had a baby after I performed surgery on her. She told me every morning when she wakes up and looks at her child, she thanks God, and then she thanks me. It is such a blessing.'

The biggest piece of advice Dr Nezhat has for people who are concerned about Asherman's is to request antibiotics after uterine issues or procedures. 'If a patient had to undergo a D&C following a miscarriage or experiences postpartum bleeding, antibiotics can help to prevent infection in the lining of the uterus,' he says. 'It is also important to look for scar tissue in the abdomen – as well as the uterus – because it is common for adhesions to be there too.'

In Australia, there are Facebook groups that provide support and information about Asherman's syndrome, as well as the website **www.ashermansaustralia.com**, which raises awareness about the condition.

Camran Nezhat, MD, FACOG, FACS
Recipient of AMA's 2020 Distinguished Service Award for Meritorious Service in the Art and Science of Medicine
Fellowship Director, Camran Nezhat Institute
Clinical Professor, University of California San Francisco (UCSF)
Adjunct Professor, University of Vienna, Austria
Former Chair, Association of Adjunct Clinical Faculty and Adjunct Clinical Professor of Surgery and OBGYN, Former Deputy Chief Department of OBGYN, Stanford University Medical Center
Director, Center for Special Minimally Invasive and Robotic Surgery
Director, Camran Nezhat Institute

A note from Paul Fisher

To men in the miscarriage trenches

By far, the hardest thing I've ever done is watch my wife struggle through recurrent miscarriages. It wasn't until we went through our first pregnancy loss that I understood how brutal the experience is. As a partner, I've felt helpless. If I could have taken away Chloe's pain, I would have. But there was nothing I could do to fix the situation or make things better. All I could do was show my support and be there for her.

Here are some lessons I've learned along the way . . .

BACK YOUR PARTNER

The biggest piece of advice I want to share to hopeful fathers is to be in your partner's corner. On this journey, my role has been to support and comfort Chloe. Whatever she needed from me, she got. If Chloe wanted to try acupuncture, I went along to the appointment with her – and even tried it myself once. I wanted to be by her side through it all. That wasn't always possible when I was on the road, but I did my best. Even when I wasn't physically next to Chloe, she knew I was there for her. I have always – and will always – have my wife's back.

LISTEN UP

In the beginning, I fell down rabbit holes on Google about miscarriage and infertility. I remember telling Chloe about all these things we should be doing and trying – as if she hadn't already researched every inch of the topic. I soon learned that wasn't helpful. There's so much misinformation out there, and so many 'helpful' people quick to tell hopeful mothers to 'just relax'. The last thing Chloe needed was me repeating nonsense to her. All it did was stress her out more.

Instead of getting lost in the noise, I started to listen to the doctors and take in as much information as I could. I listened to Chloe too, and I trusted her judgement when it came to her body. We talk about everything, and being able to communicate openly made things easier.

LEAN ON SUPPORT

The sad reality is that miscarriage is common. It happens to one in four pregnancies. When we decided to share our experiences, our friends started to open up about theirs too. It helped a lot to talk to people who understood what we were going through. Knowing we weren't alone meant a lot. I think the more we talk about hard things, the easier they are to carry. It's okay to ask for help and lean on your mates.

TAKE CARE OF YOURSELF

Having a solid routine and being active is so good for my mind and body. Chloe and I got into the habit of meditating with each other in the morning, and I really believe that's helped us. After meditating, I train and then hit the ice bath and sauna for recovery. I've been doing ice baths every day for a couple of years now, and it's done me the world of good. It never gets easier. I still have to psych myself up to get in the ice, but it's worth it. Afterward, I feel like I can tackle anything.

If you find something that works for you, stick to it. Miscarriage takes an almighty toll; you need to look after yourself to stay upright.

Eleven

A WAY FORWARD

THE NAME DR GHADIR CAME UP TWICE. HE WAS ON THE spreadsheet Erika put together for me when we first started looking into IVF in America, and he also came highly recommended by friends of ours who had conceived twins at his clinic. 'If you need an IVF doctor in the States, he's your guy,' they told us.

When I messaged Dr Ghadir, I dropped our friends' names and asked if he could give me a second opinion. He got us in for an appointment the very next day, using his lunch break to see us. Dr Ghadir's office was a breath of fresh air. He was so lovely, and we clicked straight away. I had the sense that I was exactly where I needed to be.

We did a bunch of tests and made a loose plan for next steps. Paul and I were heading to Ibiza for his 2023 residency, so we weren't going to jump into anything straight away. I wasn't going to have surgery again so soon, and I didn't have another round of IVF in me. 'Go to Europe, enjoy your summer. Just relax. I'll be here when you get back. If you need anything in the meantime, just text me,' Dr Ghadir assured us.

His words were comforting. So, too, was his parting message: 'Don't be afraid of surrogacy. It's a real option.'

And so began our surrogacy journey.

Surrogacy had been on my mind for the past two years, but I hadn't been ready to pursue it as an avenue. It wasn't until that day, sitting in agony in the LA doctor's chair with a pool of blood underneath me, that there was a shift in my mind. I had done everything in my power to try to carry my own baby – no stone had been left unturned – but it hadn't worked. I was done. I was ready to move forward.

It's strange. Even though I was looking into surrogacy and was prepared to go down that route, I still had an unshakable belief that I would have my own baby. There wasn't a bone in my body that didn't think I would give birth to a child. I was sure I was born to do it. But I was impatient. I didn't want to waste precious time continuing down the same dead-end path when there was a different path I could take – one without a dead end.

I still had two embryos in the States and three in Australia, but I wasn't going to have them transferred into my uterus if my risk of miscarrying was the same as before I'd had the Asherman's surgery. That wasn't a gamble I was willing to take. Not only because I knew I couldn't withstand another miscarriage, but also because I didn't want to waste the embryos. There was a very likely chance that if I did another egg retrieval, it might result in no embryos, like the last round of IVF I did in Australia. The embryos we had in storage were my last chance of having a baby that was genetically mine. If my uterus couldn't keep an embryo safe, I would find one that could.

As always, Paul was supportive of my choice to look into surrogacy. He was happy to follow my lead, and told me he would be in my corner no matter what.

I called my friend Lisa Messenger, the entrepreneur and author, who had been open about her own struggles with fertility. Lisa spent six years trying to have a baby herself. She did sixteen rounds of IVF, and spent more than half a million dollars in her pursuit to be a mother, before turning to surrogacy. Lisa's friend Sarah had offered to be her surrogate, and she gratefully took her up on it. Two years and two more rounds of IVF later, Sarah gave birth to baby Hugo. Lisa was a mum. Her story gave me hope.

When I called Lisa and explained my situation, she very kindly gave me the number for her surrogacy lawyer and psychologist. It was a much-needed pointer in the right direction.

I was in Greece with my sister Olivia and her then-boyfriend (now-husband) Lachie when I had a phone appointment with the lawyer. It was a bit bizarre to be having such a serious conversation in a holiday paradise, but the lawyer put me at ease right away. He explained that he'd had his own child via surrogate, so he had both lived and professional experience with the journey. He was lovely, and very thorough.

Apart from some minor logistical details, the process seemed pretty straightforward to me. I was lucky that I had already gone through IVF and so had embryos ready to go. That crossed one big thing off the list.

I had the embryos. Tick. Next up, I needed to find a surrogate. I knew where to start looking: the *Darling, Shine!* email inbox. After talking about my miscarriages so candidly on the podcast, I'd had several lovely women email offering to be my surrogate. I hadn't replied to those emails at the time, but I remembered that they were there. Part of me thought it might be strange having a listener be my surrogate, but another part told me it couldn't hurt to start with what was in front of me.

I asked my then-manager, Em, to set up initial interviews with three women who'd reached out. Em spoke to each of them, and she got a particularly good feeling from a woman named K, who lived in Queensland. 'This girl is the one,' Em told me, before organising for me and Paul to meet K over a video call as we were overseas.

Before the call, Paul and I spoke about our hopes for the person and the process. 'Do you want to get to know the surrogate and have them in our lives, or treat it like a transaction?' Paul asked. The answer was the former. Of course I wanted to have a relationship with our surrogate, the woman who was going to carry our baby. I wanted to be there for it all.

Our video call with K felt like a first date, only more intense. I was so nervous I thought I might vomit. I wanted to make a good impression. From our hotel room in London and K's home office in Queensland, we met (virtually).

'What made you think that you'd even want to do surrogacy?' I asked her.

'I've always thought that I would love to do that for someone,' K explained. 'I never really thought about doing it for a stranger. I always thought if one of my close friends or my sister couldn't conceive on their own, then I would do it for someone in my life.'

I was a stranger, but K said she felt a connection to me. She loosely knew my story from snippets I'd shared on Instagram and loved seeing us with Minnie. She saw how much Paul and I wanted to be parents, and she understood. K had three boys, and she was adamant she wasn't going to have any more children of her own. Her husband had had a vasectomy. They were done.

'I loved being pregnant, and I loved giving birth, but there's no chance of us having more kids. [Having] three boys is wild! They keep me on my toes,' K said.

'What does your husband think about your being a surrogate?' I asked.

'I only just talked to him about it, but he's cruisey,' she said, with an easy laugh. 'It's whatever I want to do with my life, we don't really hold each other back. When I make decisions, he's always on board with what I want to do.'

K was saying all the right things. We got on well, and it felt like we were on the same page.

In Australia, surrogacy can only be altruistic. Parents are not allowed to pay a surrogate for their sacrifice, time and commitment. It's a huge thing for someone to do for free. While we couldn't pay K, we could cover her medical expenses and any related travel or costs. We were up-front about wanting to take care of K in any way we could – but also very aware that we could never repay her for her generosity.

After going over the big things, we got into logistics. We asked if K would prefer giving birth in a hospital or at home, and she was open to both options. She'd had a C-section with her firstborn, and a home birth with her last-born, so she had experience with both.

K had experienced a miscarriage with her first ever pregnancy, but she was told that was quite common. She fell pregnant with her son the very next cycle and didn't have any complications. 'It was a very easy process for us,' she said.

The surrogacy lawyer had jotted down some points we should cover. Some of the questions felt strange to ask a total stranger – like if K was religious – but they were all things we needed to think about. The lawyer explained that some religions forbade abortions even on medical grounds, so if something went wrong with the pregnancy, we needed to be aware of that.

They were big topics. K and I did most of the talking. Paul sat next to me in almost total silence. 'This is the quietest I've ever been,' he said toward the end. 'I just think for someone to do this for other people is really beautiful.'

And that's when I burst into tears.

The magnitude of what K was offering to do for us was overwhelming. It was the most selfless and generous act of kindness.

We came away from the conversation with hearts full of love and hope. We decided to all take two weeks to think things over and then chat again. I knew there were lots more questions to ask and hoops to jump through, but I felt positive. For better or worse, I've always made decisions based off energy and how I feel, and I had a good feeling about K.

The lawyer said that he thinks sometimes babies born to surrogates take on some of their personality. If that is the case, we knew we would be lucky to have K as the surrogate.

There were a hundred questions in the surrogacy counselling form. Each of them had to be answered with a rating out of 'very likely', 'likely', 'neutral', 'unlikely', and 'very unlikely'. The questions covered everything from suicide ideation to travel plans and parenting style. It was in-depth and intense. And yet I felt completely at ease. I didn't have a single ounce of doubt or fear. I knew I was doing the right thing and that I was moving one step closer to having my baby. What could have been a stressful experience was just really beautiful, because the people around me made things so easy.

After our initial conversation with K, we both agreed we wanted to keep talking and move ahead with the process. We got the balls moving on the legal side and began the counselling requirements. To be able to use my embryos in Australia, Dr Ong had to do a consultation with K. He did a medical check-up with her and got a feel for her as a person. From there, Dr Ong took our case for surrogacy to the board of his clinic, and our request was approved. K could use my embryos.

It felt like a milestone.

For the first time in a long time, I felt like I could relax knowing that the wheels were in motion. It was exciting to know we were making progress toward our dream. I was at peace with the decisions we'd made in the past, and with our plan for the future. It probably helped that we were in Ibiza, a place we love so much.

For the second time in as many years, we were spending the Euro summer with Ell and Minnie, who was nearly two and such a cheeky cutie. When they landed in Ibiza, it had been several months since we'd seen each other, and I had missed them terribly. We jumped straight into our Ibiza tradition and took Minnie to Fish Shack restaurant on the beach for a swim in the ocean and her favourite lamb cutlets.

I loved Minnie so much; it was painful to be away from her. She grew so quickly – too quickly! I didn't want to miss a second of it.

Revealing questions to ask a potential surrogate

There are so many things to consider and questions to ask when speaking to a potential surrogate. Of course, there are medical questions to cover: how many pregnancies have you had? Did you have any complications? Do you have a history of miscarriage? Are there any genetic conditions in your family? How is your current health condition? Are you taking any medication? How do you feel about necessary prenatal testing?

Then there are the lifestyle questions: do you smoke or drink? How often do you exercise? Are you willing to adjust your exercise routine during pregnancy? How would you describe your diet?

And the all-important legal questions: do you understand the legal implications of surrogacy? Do you have a legal representative or are you willing to get one? Are you comfortable with the legal contracts involved in surrogacy?

Logistical questions are important. So, too, are more personal questions about the potential surrogate, their life and interests. Here is a list we prepared earlier . . .

- What are the three biggest things that influenced your decision to be a surrogate?
- How would you describe your relationship with your family? And what do they think about your decision to be a surrogate?
- What are your three main concerns about the surrogacy process?

- What level of communication would you like throughout the journey?
- What does an average day in your life look like?
- How would your best friend describe you?
- What was the last book you read?
- What was your favourite subject in school and why?
- How do you like to unwind after a big week?
- What do you want to know about us as intended parents?
- What would you like us to tell our child about you as they get older?

Twelve

A CURVEBALL

Seeing Paul reunite with Minnie after so many months apart was epic. They have an unbreakable bond. At that age, she was obsessed with him, and the feeling was mutual. They bounced off each other, like the little kids they both were at heart. Watching Paul carrying Minnie on his shoulders, I knew he was going to be an amazing dad. Not that he was trying to be a dad to Minnie! Chumpy would always be her dad. But Paul loved and cared for Minnie like she was his own.

When Paul talked about the kind of father he wanted to be, he said he wanted to be present, to be fun and to give his child the very best upbringing. He was already doing all of those things with Minnie. We felt so lucky to have her and Ell in our lives.

In the two years since we launched *Darling, Shine!*, the podcast grew bigger than we could ever have imagined. We hit a million listens during the second series, and hosted a big party with all our mates on Pittwater to celebrate. From there, the momentum didn't stop. I know a lot of podcasters say this, but our listeners became a real community. We started a private Facebook group where members share their own stories, ask for advice and offer support. It was beautiful to see such a sisterhood grow out of me and Ell talking shit with each other. Paul came home from a gig one night and (half-jokingly) had the shits. A group of girls had told him they'd only come to the show to see me, and they were upset when I wasn't there. 'Tell your wife we love her,' they said.

In Ibiza, we were all feeling the love. Just like we'd done the year before, we took a boat out to Es Vedrà and had a magical day on the water. In the time between Es Vedrà trips, I had gone through an unsuccessful embryo transfer, an unsuccessful egg retrieval, a brutal miscarriage (my fourth) and an invasive surgery. I had endured some of my darkest days – days that nearly broke me – and had changed as a person. I'm sure part of me was more jaded and cynical about the world, but a bigger part of me remained hopeful. I'd taken blow after blow, but I was still standing, and Paul was right there by my side.

Watching the sun set over the Mediterranean Sea one night, I made a wish. I told my baby I was ready for her. In my mind, she was a girl. I don't know why; all five of the babies I had lost were boys.

Santa Monica is 9808 kilometres from Ibiza. It was a distance I was willing to travel to experience the Panchakarma Retreat at Surya Spa. The retreat is run by Martha Soffer, who is regarded as the Ayurvedic Healer to the Stars. People literally fly from all over the world for treatments with her – I'm one of them. I saw someone post about Surya Spa on Instagram, and I knew that Martha had worked with Kourtney Kardashian and Travis Barker on their fertility journey. I wanted in.

So many people don't get the opportunity to do a retreat like this, and I'm so grateful I could.

Before arriving at the retreat, I started a pre-cleanse, taking increasing teaspoons of ghee every day. I also stopped drinking to prepare my body for what was to come. Panchakarma was described as a 'reset', and it felt like exactly what I needed. I was ready to detox.

On day one, I met Martha, who I swear glowed. I didn't tell Martha why I was at the retreat or what I had been through. I didn't need to. Martha inspected my tongue, looked into my eyes and took my pulse. From that, she was able to tell me exactly what was going on and exactly why I was there. It was extraordinary. Martha discovered there was a combination of damp and heat in my body, which needed balancing out. She put a treatment plan together to 'warm up my oven' and 'remove my sluggishness'.

I was astounded by Martha's knowledge and wisdom. The week-long retreat included daily Ayurvedic treatments using personalised herbal oils, which 'restore mind, body and spirit'. Every morning began with a two-hour, four-handed massage. It was heaven. Mostly. Some days I felt agitated and couldn't relax, other days I melted completely.

Each day, we had the same thing for lunch: mung beans, rice and vegetables. I thought I would get bored eating the same thing, but I ended up craving it. As well as the Ayurvedic treatments, I did private yoga classes and breathwork sessions. Paul had never done breathwork before and was super interested in trying it, so he joined me for that session at the end of the retreat. We lay on mats next to each other and were guided through the process. This might sound like I'm exaggerating, but it was a euphoric experience. We randomly had a giggle fit right in the middle of it. The energy in the room was next level. While we were still lying down, I had an overwhelming urge to hold Paul's hand. When we eventually sat up, we shared our experiences. 'It's so weird, but I really wanted to hold your hand at the end,' Paul said.

We'd had the same thought at the same time. I think Paul and I are always very connected, but after the breathwork session, there was so much love, gratitude and compassion between us. I felt so unbelievably happy. On my last day at the retreat, Martha gave me a hand-blended oil with instructions to put a drop in my bellybutton every day. 'The bellybutton is connected to life,' she said, explaining that the oil would help me call on the energy to fall pregnant.

After five days at Surya, I genuinely felt like I was floating. I returned to Ibiza with Paul feeling freer than I had in years. It wasn't just the retreat; it was the plan we had in place. I knew when Paul finished his residency in Ibiza, I would head back to Australia to meet K and her husband in person and start the physical surrogacy process. We had completed all the legal and counselling requirements and were ready to dive in the deep end together. It was happening.

But first, Paul and I were finally going to have a honeymoon. We hadn't been able to go away after our wedding in 2020, because the world went into lockdown, so we decided to take the opportunity at last. We booked a holiday to the Maldives, just the two of us.

Our hotel was the definition of paradise. We had an overwater villa above the most crystal-clear sea I've ever seen. It was so beautiful it made me want to cry.

The trip was exactly what we both needed. It rained a lot of the time we were there, which forced us both to really slow down and stop. We spent hours in our room together, talking and giggling, and reading *The 5 Love Languages* by Gary Chapman. Paul and I had been together for eleven years, but it felt like we were getting to know each other on an even deeper level. Our true colours certainly came out while we were playing UNO . . .

There's this meme that's painfully true: 'The person you become when playing UNO is who you really are.' As it goes, I'm a stickler for the rules, and slightly competitive. Meanwhile, Paul is cheeky and forever trying his luck. Who knew?

Apart from the UNO wars, our time huddled up in the villa was like being in a little love bubble. It almost felt like our early days staying in the front room of my parents' house and cherishing every minute together. Except, obviously, the Maldives was a lot more luxurious.

Paul joined me on my break from drinking. We'd never been huge drinkers anyway, but we were trying to get into a healthy routine, and that was part of it. We were both in good physical shape – and that helped with our mental shape. Knowing we were going back to Australia to begin the surrogacy journey took so much pressure off my shoulders. It felt like we could breathe.

After our honeymoon, we spent a week in Bali, then I returned to Australia while Paul went back to Europe for a few shows. Everything had been green-lit for the surrogacy process to begin. K and her husband had signed the official surrogacy agreement, and we were going to sign the hard copy when Paul got home. In the meantime, I was going to meet with K and her husband in Brisbane ahead of the first transfer the following month. It was go time. Bring it on.

I had mentally prepared myself for the surrogacy process, but nothing could have prepared me for the spanner the universe threw in the works.

The day after I got home from Bali, I had an appointment booked for a doctor to perform a sonohysterogram on me, to get a clear picture of the scar tissue in my uterus. Even though I wasn't going to do IVF again (for the foreseeable future), I still wanted to get to the bottom of what was happening inside me. I'd left my last appointment with that doctor in LA feeling shattered and lost. I was haunted by the sight of the blood on the floor underneath me after the doctor attempted to remove the remaining scar tissue with saline, and wanted to get a second medical opinion following the Asherman's surgery.

Ellidy was picking me up to take me to the appointment. While I waited for her to arrive, I read over the pre-procedure notes. One of the notes said 'abstain from sexual activity in the lead-up to the procedure'. Oops. I obviously hadn't done that – I was on my honeymoon! – so I decided to do a quick pregnancy test to be sure.

A faint line appeared. I was pregnant.

I called Ell straight away. 'Uh, slight change of plans, sis.'

I bought my fifth pregnancy journal. On the first page, I wrote, in gold pen: 'Date found out: 13/10/23. The day after I got home from Bali and Maldives from our honeymoon. Booked in for procedure and took pregnancy test just in case 🖤'

I was overjoyed. And fucking terrified. The LA doctor's parting words replayed in my head: 'Don't try and fall pregnant again, because if you do, you will miscarry.'

I'd never wanted anyone to be wrong more than them.

After Ell, I called Dr Ong. Even though it wasn't an IVF pregnancy, I instinctively called to tell him I was pregnant. He was my safe person. 'Come straight in, we'll do blood tests,' he said.

The tests confirmed my pregnancy. Dr Ong was thrilled for us. 'How fantastic,' he said. 'Whenever pregnancy happens, we need to embrace it and give it the best chance.' I was put on Clexane, prednisone, progesterone and aspirin.

I was three-and-a-half-weeks pregnant. Paul and I had conceived naturally on our honeymoon, just like my parents had thirty-two years earlier. I'd thought I was going to have a honeymoon baby when I got pregnant the day after our wedding. But it turned out, I was having a honeymoon baby after our official honeymoon. I had only fallen pregnant naturally twice; once after the wedding in 2020, and then on our belated honeymoon in 2023.

It felt like our baby had been waiting for the exact right moment to come along. I always hated it when people told me, 'just relax and it'll happen,' but it kills me to say that in our case, that is exactly what happened.

Paul was on his way back to the States from Spain, where he'd done a couple of shows to close the Euro summer season. He was heading to LA for one of the biggest shows of his career. The party and event brand he'd founded with his good friend Chris Lake, Under Construction, was putting on a world-first gig. The boys were shutting down Hollywood Boulevard for an epic block party. It had never been done before. They were creating LA history.

Paul was in the lounge at Madrid Airport with his best mate, Little Fritter (real name Kane), when I called him. I tried to keep the chat casual, but he knew straight away that something was up.

'I've got something to tell you,' I said. 'I'm pregnant.'

'What do you mean you're pregnant?' he asked me, unable to fathom what I'd just said.

'I just took a test and I'm pregnant,' I repeated.

I could almost hear the cogs turning in his brain. I knew exactly how he felt, I think I was still in shock myself. The positive test had given me whiplash. I'd been racing ahead in one direction – toward surrogacy – when suddenly I was stopped in my tracks and turned around. The disbelief was real.

When Paul got off the phone, he turned to Kane and told him the news. 'Chloe's pregnant.' They were both so stoked and couldn't stop smiling. But under Paul's smile, there was worry, too. He didn't want to get his hopes up. We'd been here before, and we knew how quickly 'stoked' could turn into 'shattered'. Paul wrote a note right then and there in the airport lounge. 'Please let this be. Please universe, don't be so cruel and take this away. Please let us have this baby,' he wished.

On the Gold Coast, I was saying my own silent prayers. I was so scared to lose the miracle baby inside me, but the fear was slightly softened by the knowledge of our back-up plan. If the worst was to happen, I knew we could start surrogacy straight away. K was good to go.

I broke the news to her in person. We had already planned to meet in Brisbane the week after I got back to Australia. I booked a room for her and her husband, and another for me and Ell, at The Calile Hotel on James Street in Fortitude Valley. Paul was still away, so Ell was my support person. I remember the elevator trip from our hotel room down to the restaurant in vivid detail. The gold doors, the travertine floor, the shiny buttons. I took it all in.

I was so nervous about meeting K for the first time in person and giving her this unexpected update, I thought I might be sick. But the anxious nausea lifted the moment I met K. She was just as warm and personable in real life as she had been over our video-call.

When I told K we would have to press pause on the surrogacy plans because – surprise! – I was pregnant, she was nothing but happy for us. I'm sure there might have been some slight disappointment because we'd already put so much time into the process, but she completely understood. I was quick to assure her that we'd be in touch if things didn't work out, which I knew was a very real possibility, but I was praying this time would be different.

Affirmations to write down and repeat

Today is the start of our journey.

The universe is on our side.

I am healthy, my eggs are healthy.

My body is fertile and ready.

I am so grateful for what my body can do.

Patience and care help me prepare.

My eggs are developing exactly as they should be.

I have never been more ready to meet you, my precious little rainbow baby.

I trust in the divine timing for us.

I will not push my limits, and I will be soft and kind to myself.

I will take each day as it comes and remember to breathe.

Helpful books to read (or flick through)

The fertility journey is a vulnerable one. I would have bought anything, tried anything and read anything if it increased my chances of falling pregnant. Logically, I know there's no magic pill to have a baby – trust me, if there was, I would have found it. But there's still a part of me that keeps looking for one. I bought so many books, joined so many Facebook groups and listened to so many podcast episodes while trying to conceive. Some of the books sat on my shelf unopened. These are the ones I picked up and drew inspiration from . . .

It Starts with the Egg by Rebecca Fett

This book explores how the science of egg quality can help you get pregnant naturally, prevent miscarriage and improve your odds in IVF. A step-by-step guide to taking back control, using the latest research to go from feeling powerless to being informed and proactive.

Empowered Fertility: A Practical Twelve-Step Guide by Claire Hall with Dr Devora Lieberman

A helpful resource for navigating infertility by a Sydney-based life coach and counsellor and fertility expert. The steps include 'Accepting what is', 'Releasing control' and 'Building your emotional toolkit'. All very relevant and necessary skills.

***Fertility Breakthrough* by Gabriela Rosa**

This book is thick with science, research and personal experience, from the world-renowned fertility specialist Gabriela Rosa. There are chapters on misconceptions, common mistakes, dietary choices and the pillars of fertility, as well as 'prescriptions' for a fertility reset. I highlighted so many passages; every other page is stained with fluoro ink. This is one I kept coming back to: 'When a body is out of balance stress directly impacts its hormones and reproductive organs. It increases the production of cortisol, adrenaline and noradrenaline – also known as stress hormones. The problem with this increase in stress hormone production is that reproductive hormones are made from the same precursor: pregnenolone . . . High levels of stress hormones are associated with weight gain, infertility and miscarriage.'

***The Ayurvedic Guide to Fertility* by Heather Grzych**

You already know I'm a big fan of Ayurvedic treatments, and this book contains plenty of the ancient 'science of life'. It's 'a practical, intentional guide to creating enhanced conditions for conception'. Woo-woo? A little. Fascinating? A lot. The chapter on 'The Four Fertility Factors' – seed, season, field and water – was particularly interesting.

Thirteen

WHATEVER WILL BE

THE MORNING SICKNESS FELT LIKE A HANGOVER, WHICH WAS ironic, because I was completely sober. For obvious reasons.

I remember turning up at Ell's house one morning in my first trimester, desperately trying not to spew. 'I love being pregnant, I love being pregnant, I love being pregnant,' I repeated like a mantra. It was true – I loved it – but that didn't mean it was easy.

After my miscarriages, I promised myself I wouldn't complain about being pregnant if I was lucky enough to experience it again. Morning sickness? Bring it on. Stretch marks? Go ahead. Reflux? Game on. I wanted to cherish every moment.

Actually, if I'm honest, I could've done without the indigestion. It felt like I had a permanent fire roaring in the back of my throat. I was burping like I've never burped before. I drove around with a bottle of Gaviscon in the car and drank it like it was water.

I had my first scan at six-and-a-half weeks in early November. Paul was still away, so Ell was my support person. She was scared for me, I could tell. She had seen me get excited over positive pregnancy tests before, only for it to end in tears. I don't think Ell believed that the baby was real until she saw the heartbeat on the screen. It was such a special experience to share.

Early on in the pregnancy, I had some spotting, and I immediately thought the worst. I couldn't handle the prospect of losing another baby, and yet, the thought consumed me. I was petrified, and then anxious about being petrified. It was a vicious cycle. Long after my spotting stopped, I still checked for blood every time I went to the bathroom.

Paul was home for our ten-week scan. At the appointment, I could tell our ultrasound tech, Bec, was crossing her fingers for us. She knew our story, so I'm sure she was holding her breath just like I was. When we saw the baby moving around, we all let out a collective sigh of relief. The baby looked like it was waving and kicking its legs. It was real, and it was alive.

We tentatively started telling the people closest to us. However, I didn't buy anything for the baby; I didn't religiously write in my pregnancy journal; I didn't take polaroids every week as I had done in the past. I didn't want to jinx anything, even though I knew that wasn't a logical thought.

I decided I wasn't going to walk on eggshells. My feet were sore from all the tiptoeing I'd done over the years. I made a promise to myself that I wouldn't obsess over this pregnancy in the same way I had with my others. I wanted to let go of the stress and surrender to the universe. I kept telling myself: 'Whatever will be, will be. Your story is already written.'

Paul was heading off on an Asian tour, starting in Japan, and I went with him as planned. My mum was worried it was a bad idea; she thought I should stay home and rest. But I was adamant. 'I'm not going to sit at home and hope for the best. If I'm going to have a miscarriage, it's going to happen wherever I am. There's nothing I can do to change that.'

I highlighted a passage in the fertility book I was reading, *Fertility Breakthrough* by Gabriela Rosa: 'Choose right now to stop being the victim in a life that hasn't yet turned out how you want it to – and take charge. It begins with you and ends with you . . . If you can't be happy with what you already have, right now, you never will.'

Oof, those words cut straight to the bone. I took them to heart and vowed to try to be happy in the present; to focus on what I did have instead of what I was missing; to keep living my life.

When we landed in Tokyo, I knew immediately I had made the right decision. It's such a cool city, and we had a fun trip in store. Paul's shows at Raise Nightclub were sensational. I was grateful to be there with him, even though I didn't go to the club.

Don't get me wrong, I was still experiencing first trimester nausea and indigestion, but I was glad to be gassy in Japan. More than anything, I was glad to be with Paul. He couldn't stop touching my belly. His hands kept gravitating to it. I don't know if he was feeling it to make sure the baby was real or willing it to stay where it was.

The baby was real, and it was staying put. We gave it two nicknames: Bubba Fish and Coco Baby.

I saw my baby before I met her. Yes, she was a girl in the vision. I was doing a spirit baby session with a medium named Avalon at the end of 2020. While she spoke and chanted to me, I went into a sort of vortex. That's where I saw my daughter. She had my skin – golden olive – and Paul's eyes – bright blue. The little girl was playing in a field. I wanted more than anything to meet her, and I had a steadfast belief that I would.

I had seen so many psychics on my fertility journey, and before that, too. I was usually in a state of flux when I booked an appointment. Whether you believe in psychics or not, there's a comfort in getting guidance from a higher place. I remember having a session with psychic medium Rebecca Mayhew in

2012, just after I met Paul in Bali. She told me I was going to meet a guy, *the* guy. She said he had a big personality, that he was going to be super successful and that we were going to have houses all around the world. Paul only ticked one of those boxes; he was a character, but he was a broke surfer who couldn't afford one mortgage, let alone multiple. He was the guy for me, so I figured, as far as Rebecca went, one out of three wasn't bad. I'd rather have just the good guy any day.

It turned out he was a three-for-three. We didn't buy our first home in Palm Beach until 2020. It was only afterward that we bought places in LA, Ibiza and Bali. Almost a decade after my reading with Rebecca, I realised she had been talking about Paul all along.

It was always him. And now we were pregnant again.

My belly popped quite early, at around the twelve-week mark. I hadn't truly experienced having a baby belly, so that was confirmation that this pregnancy wasn't the same as the others. We had a chance. That bump restored my faith in miracles.

Every day, I would look at my pregnant body in the mirror and take it all in. I know it's a cliché, but the female body truly is extraordinary. Creating life felt magical. I stared at my reflection and applauded myself on growing the little human inside me: 'Wow, congratulations, you're doing it.'

I remember going for a swim at the beach and feeling so proud of my belly. I was even proud of all the bruises on it from the clexane injections, because they were a part of the story. My story. For four and a half years, my tummy had been covered in bruises from IVF injections, and I finally had something to show for it, even though we hadn't fallen pregnant using IVF.

On Christmas Day 2023, we announced our pregnancy publicly on Instagram. 'The greatest gift of all 🖤 I've waited my whole life for you,' I wrote. 'The most wanted and loved baby Fisher will be joining the tour in 2024. We are still pinching ourselves that we've finally been chosen to become parents.

'Although this post is the single most happiest moment in my life, I know how incredibly hard announcements like these are for those struggling with infertility,' I continued. 'After four years of trying to conceive, thousands of needles, eight rounds of IVF, multiple surgeries, I've lived this nightmare. I know this pain and suffering all too well, no-one deserves to endure this feeling. I feel you all, I see you all and I completely understand the disappointment and sadness you are all feeling. Please stay positive and manifest your healthy baby. I pray you hold your miracle in your arms soon. My heart is with you.'

As soon as the post went up, I had to put my phone away. There were hundreds of thousands of likes, thousands of comments, and hundreds of private messages. It was beautiful; so many people were over the moon for us. A lot of them wrote about how they burst into tears for us when they saw the news. I couldn't believe how many people cared so much and were so invested in our journey to parenthood. It was beyond touching. The positive energy surrounded and encompassed us. There was nowhere else I wanted to be.

I asked my mum to tell me my birth story. I'd heard it before over the years, but I wanted to hear it again. The way Mum tells it, I didn't have the easiest arrival into the world. She had a long labour and was eventually induced. That was a worry for her, because her family has a history of blood clots. During labour, I was digging into my mum's pelvic bone and refusing to come out, so they had to use forceps. I was born at 11.10 pm, weighing seven pounds and eleven ounces, with forceps marks on my head.

That number was so close to the one I'd had tattooed on my arm in honour of my grandma – 11:11. I said a silent prayer to Grandma, Poppa and Chumpy in the sky, asking them to keep this baby safe.

After having a family Christmas on the Gold Coast, we headed over to LA for a US stint. I ushered in the New Year backstage at Paul's gig, sitting on the couch, doing puzzles and eating pizza with Tallara. I wore a sheer top with my little belly poking out. Everyone kept giving me a tummy rub, like

I was a good luck Buddha. When Paul came off stage, I gave him the biggest hug. We both welcomed 2024 knowing – hoping – it would be the year we held our baby in our arms.

I had tunnel vision. I was so focused on growing the baby inside me, I shut out other parts of my life. I'm not using that as an excuse for what I'm about to tell you, but I'm sure it played a part.

At the start of 2024, Ellidy decided she was going to sell her house and buy a new place, somewhere smaller, more manageable and closer to the beach. It was a big deal. When Chumpy died, Ell made a promise to herself that she would do whatever it took to keep the house – Chumpy's house, their house. All of her last memories with him were in that home; in the music room downstairs where he spent hours making magic, in the pool that he kept sparkling clean, and in the pantry, which held a gluten-free chocolate cake mix that he'd bought the last time they did a grocery shop together.

Ell had worked her arse off to keep the house and pay the mortgage – for her, Minnie and Rummi – but she was struggling to keep up with the maintenance. She knew Chumpy would be looking down on her and begging her to water the garden or clean the pool. She hated the idea of disappointing him. For that reason and others, she decided to sell, and she found a place she wanted to buy. It was a real fixer-upper, but right on the beach, and perfect for her. To make it happen, she needed a sum of money to get the number across the line.

Ell was super casual when she brought it up with me. 'Hey sis, my accountant said I need this extra sum of money,' she said. 'I know we have the money in the business account, can I grab it out?'

I answered as a business partner instead of as a friend. 'Yes, you can, let's just speak to the accountant to make sure the cashflow is fine and that our forecast for the year allows it,' I replied.

What I didn't know at the time – namely because Ell hadn't communicated this to me – was how tough things were for her. She was a single mum, juggling a business, bills and a property sale and purchase. It was all too much. Ell snapped. She left me a voice message saying I had no fucking idea how hard it was for her. And she was right! I didn't know, because she didn't talk about it. Had I known how stressed she was, I would have transferred the money from my personal account. The whole thing came down to a lack of communication, but it ended with a blow-up.

Ell and I didn't speak to each other for a week. I cried every day. I swear, fighting with your bestie can be more brutal than fighting with your husband. The silence was cutting. Even though Ell and I are different in most ways, we have one thing in common: we're both as stubborn as each other. Neither one of us was going to be the first to reach out.

As it went, it was *Darling, Shine!* that brought us back together. We had a planning meeting about the fifth season of the podcast, and the day before the meeting, I flat-out said I wouldn't go unless Ell called me beforehand. My phone didn't ring until an hour before the scheduled meeting. On the call, we each talked and we each listened. And we cried. I saw where she was coming from, and she saw where I was coming from. Communicating cleared the air. Funny that.

At the end of the day, I have so much love and respect for Ell, and I know she has the same for me. She is my friend, my business partner and my chosen family. I think it's because of how close we are that we can fight the way we do. We have disagreements – usually because of the aforementioned lack of communication – but we always sort them out and come away stronger for it. There's a reason I call Ell 'sis', and it's not just because we fight like sisters. No matter how big the tiff, we will always be there for each other.

By the end of January 2024, Ell and I were back to our usual selves, annoying each other, but loving each other more. In the first episode of *Darling, Shine!* for the year, we set our intentions for the next twelve months. Ell said she wanted to improve on communicating. 'I want to be able to talk about serious things, and the things that I'm struggling with. Sometimes I just try to deal with everything on my own,' she said. 'I want to be a big girl and have big girl chats, and that means being open with people and telling them if I have a problem.'

In a later episode, I told Ell exactly how I felt about her. 'Can I just give a shout-out to this chick? This is a single mum who's absolutely worked her bloody arse off the last three years supporting her little family. You are the most generous and kindest person,' I said when she announced she had finalised her house purchase. 'Being able to purchase something on your own as a single woman is amazing. You should be so proud of yourself, Ell.'

Luckily we were in a good place, because Ell and I were off to Eden Health Retreat in the Currumbin Valley for three nights together. When we booked it, we didn't really clock the word 'Health' in the title – we were focused on the 'Retreat' part. We imagined daily massages, gourmet meals and gentle yoga classes. We didn't realise there was no sugar, no caffeine, no salt or pepper and no wine (for Ell). After our first dinner of steak, broccoli and potato (cooked in coconut oil, sans all seasoning and sauce), I was ecstatic to find a Twirl chocolate bar in my bag.

Apart from the smuggled chocolate, Ell and I committed to the retreat. Well, we tried to. I did a stretch class, an acupuncture session and a nutrition talk, while Ell did a boxing class, a sauna session and a mud bath. Somehow, we missed the sweet-potato brownie at morning tea, and we were both devastated. Ell used my pregnancy to try to get us extra food at lunch.

I know I'm focusing a lot on the food, or lack thereof, but food really is the bond that anchors my and Ell's friendship. We think about food 24/7. We love nothing more than imagining our next meal and then getting to eat that meal.

The best part of the whole retreat was Ell getting to feel the baby kick for the first time.

After Eden, we went home to the Gold Coast, where Paul and I were booked in for our twenty-week scan. It felt like another landmark on the list of milestones we were crossing off: the twelve-week mark, the furthest we'd been in a pregnancy, the belly pop, and now the twenty-week scan. It was during that scan that the reality of the pregnancy started to sink in. The baby was growing and meeting all the recommended markers, Bec explained.

We didn't want to know the sex of the baby, so I looked away when Bec got to that part. 'I don't know how I'll cope if it's a girl, I'll be way too excited,' I said to Bec, niggling for clues. 'But I think it'll be a boy.' Somehow, Bec kept a straight face the whole time. She didn't give anything away.

Of course, everyone says they don't care about gender, they only care that the baby is healthy. That's true! Still, I dreamed about having a little girl, the one from my vision.

'It's starting to feel so real,' I wrote in my pregnancy journal. 'I can't seem to work out if it's a boy or a girl from the scans. Some angles it looks like a little girl, others a little boy. Cute little cheeks like Mummy.'

The several plastic sharps disposal containers were all full. I wanted to count the number of needles I'd injected in the last three and a half years during IVF, so I collected all the boxes from LA and Australia. We wanted to do a guessing game, like count the jelly beans in the jar. We never got the final answer though; we couldn't get the containers open. They were simply too full, too tight, too stuck.

I still think about getting a hacksaw and cracking them open, but maybe some things are better left alone. Maybe I don't need to look at the needles again; maybe I don't need to know the number of injections.

I was in the early stages of my pregnancy when I went to my first in-person board meeting for The Pink Elephants Support Network, who do the most amazing work in the miscarriage space. I had been approached by the founder, Samantha Payne, in mid-2023, while I was in Ibiza, inviting me to join the board of the organisation she'd started in 2016 to provide much-needed – and at the time, non-existent – support. In the time since, Pink Elephants has become a vital resource for those impacted by early pregnancy loss. I was so proud to join Sam and the team on their mission.

Of course, I had lived experience of miscarriage to bring to the table, but I also had business, marketing and digital knowledge that I thought could help build the organisation.

Knowing how important the work was, I wanted to make a serious contribution. In 2024, *Darling, Shine!* chose Pink Elephants as our charity of the year and we released a special cap with 'Lil Darlins' embroidered on the front and a small pink elephant on the side. The idea was for those who've experienced pregnancy loss to wear the cap and start conversations, and for loved ones to buy a cap to show their support. We ended up raising $40,000 for the cause, which was huge.

It was complicated to be doing so much work in the miscarriage space while pregnant. I felt a sense of guilt. I knew the sharp sting that bump shots delivered to hopeful parents. I hated the idea of rubbing my miracle in the face of someone waiting for theirs, even unintentionally. I pulled back from sharing on social media because I didn't want to be triggering.

It was a fine line to tread. On one side, I wanted to keep sharing my life for everyone who was invested or interested or looking for some hope. On the other, I wanted to keep my pregnancy to myself to protect anyone who might be hurt by it. I walked that line as best I could, but I'm sure I made missteps along the way. My bump continued to grow.

Fourteen

INDEFINITELY

I KNEW PREGNANCY WOULD BE AMAZING, BUT IT WAS EVEN better than I expected.

The longer my pregnancy went on, the more settled I felt. When the baby started to kick around the twenty-week mark, it was so incredibly reassuring. Feeling it wriggle and hiccup gave me a sense of peace. Even when the baby kicked off as soon as I went to bed at night, after being still all day. Cheeky baby. I didn't care. If it was moving, it was alive.

With the reassurance of its movement, the baby, Paul and I travelled over to Bali for our annual 'family vacay' with Ell and Minnie, and our close mates Richie and Jaynee. We stayed at our fave spot in Uluwatu, where a year earlier I'd been recovering from my fourth miscarriage. To be back in

Bali with a baby bump was pretty emotional. My belly was growing rapidly, and it felt really tight.

On 6 March, I wrote in my pregnancy journal 'How can I get bigger than this? I can't even begin to imagine how tight and uncomfortable I'm going to be closer to my due date.'

Later that month, I joined Paul in the States for a string of shows. He was set to play the iconic Ultra Music Festival in Miami. It was a huge deal – he was headlining with Chris Lake – and he was chomping at the bit. It was raining, but that didn't dampen Paul's excitement . . . until it did. The rain became torrential. Then the thunder and lightning hit.

We were on a boat, waiting to be dropped off at the stage area for Paul's set when the festival was evacuated. A flash flood ripped through the venue. The water and the lightning weren't a good fit with a big crowd and all the electronics. The risk of electrocution was too high, and the event had to be cancelled. Paul was gutted. He and Chris had worked so hard to get to that position, and for it to be washed out was actually crushing. Normally the boys might have gone for a drink to commiserate, but Paul was too rattled to even do that. It was a quiet trip back to our hotel.

We didn't have time to sit with our feelings, though. A day later, Paul played Club Space, also in Miami, which is a 24/7 nonstop party. His set went from 4 am to 11 am, and I decided to check it out for an hour or so, after my morning coffee at the hotel. I got up at 6 am, did my make-up and put on a tight little white lace mini that showed off my bump. While I was grabbing my coffee, I ran into our friend Ian, who had been up all night at the club and was sneaking back to the hotel to get some rest. When I told him I was heading in for Paul's set, he paused, then said, 'Ah, fuck it. I'm going to come back with you, let's do it.'

When we arrived at Space, the security helped me through the crowd to the stage. I felt like Moses parting the sea. As I walked through the hordes of people, I felt all their eyes on me. I was sober, relatively well-rested and clearly quite pregnant. Meanwhile, everyone else had been up all night raving. Some people weren't quite on Earth, they were on a higher plane. They looked at me, then at my belly, then back at me. I could tell they were struggling to comprehend what they were seeing. I wonder if some thought they were hallucinating, probably thinking, *What is a pregnant lady doing here at this hour?* It was such a classic. I'm sure I rattled some people that day. I drew such a sense of power from my baby belly.

I danced along to Paul's set and hoped the baby could hear its dad in his element. No doubt the baby was sleeping though. C'est la vie.

Back in LA, my US friends hosted the most beautiful baby shower for me in March. I wore a sheer, long-sleeved, white lace gown, a floral lei and a flower crown. During the intimate lunch, my friend Daisy, who is a breathwork and meditation teacher and also the wife of Paul's publicist, James, led a mother's blessing.

'I remember the first time I met Chloe at a dinner with her, Paul and James,' Daisy said to the group. 'I was having a shit day, working in a gnarly job and feeling stressed. I really didn't want to go to this dinner, but I did. Chloe didn't know any of that when she sat down across from me and gave me the biggest smile. Her smile brought so much love and happiness to me, and it turned my whole day around. Since that day, I've always had a spot for you, Chloe, in my heart.'

It was the sweetest memory for her to share, and it genuinely brought me to tears. After that, Daisy gave everyone a candle and asked them to write a hope and intention for me and the baby on it. The idea was for the girls to light their candles when I went into labour and to send me energy and strength from afar. Some of the intentions included 'miracles', 'strength' and 'warmth'. The idea of having candles lit for me around the world was so heartwarming.

The girls also had a brilliant t-shirt made for me. It was designed to look like a band tour tee, and it listed all the places I'd travelled to while I was pregnant, from the Maldives to Tokyo, Tulum to Miami.

After the baby shower, Paul and I put the finishing touches on the nursery in our LA home. We bought a change table, cot and bouncer, built the pram and Paul tested out the rocking chair. The baby had been blessed with so many great books, cute teddies and a lush Gucci baby blanket.

This was our fifth pregnancy, but our first time setting up a nursery. It was beautiful, but bittersweet. I thought about all the babies who I didn't get to bring home from the hospital, and all the empty pages in their pregnancy journals. I rubbed my belly and felt immense gratitude for it.

After a month in the States, I returned to Australia in April for the imminent arrival of our bundle of joy. On the Goldy, Paul and I did a hypnobirthing course together over two days. Part of it involved staring into each other's eyes for three minutes. It was weirdly beautiful and unexpectedly emotional for me; I couldn't stop crying. I swear all the pregnancy hormones must have hit me at once.

I've always loved Paul's eyes, and in that moment, they said so much. 'We've got this, babe, it's happening, just like we always knew it would. Our baby is on its way,' he said without speaking.

The ocean soothed my aching body. It was June, the start of winter, but the sun was out, and the water was warm on the Gold Coast. I lowered my enormous belly into the sea and let the salt water hold me. Pure bliss.

I needed the relief. I was huge, heavy and uncomfortable. My bladder ached because the baby was putting so much pressure on it. I could barely walk up stairs or roll over in bed. I figured that was all normal for that stage of pregnancy, but because I'd never been at that point before, I had no way of knowing. My due date was 26 June, but I couldn't imagine getting any bigger than I was.

On 30 April 2024, I had gone for a routine thirty-two-week scan at the ultrasound clinic to measure the baby and see how they were tracking. The baby was super healthy and weighing in above average. I was stoked.

But that's when things took a turn. The sonographer measured my cervix and found that it had shortened quite substantially, and was opening at the top. That's exactly what happens before you go into labour. But I was only thirty-two weeks – more than a month away from my due date. It was too soon.

I didn't have a hospital bag packed. The nursery was nowhere near ready.

I was sent from the ultrasound clinic straight to my obstetrician. Thankfully, they were in the same building and right outside the hospital. 'Right, we're sending you to the hospital. You've got to go on bed rest. We don't want the baby coming this early. We need it to keep cooking,' my obstetrician told me. To bed, I went. I wanted to be on the safe side more than anyone.

My obstetrician took a swab, which could apparently tell if I would go into labour in the next twenty-four hours. Thankfully, the swab said no. Still, the hospital was where I needed to be. I went to John Flynn Hospital on the Gold Coast and was initially taken straight to the birthing suite, but soon put in a suite in the maternity ward.

I would be there indefinitely. My shortened cervix was a concern, so too was the excess fluid I was carrying. I was given a steroid shot to help the baby's lungs develop. I took solace in the knowledge that if the baby was born a month early, it would more than likely be okay. But still, I hoped it would stay put for a little while longer.

The objective was to get to (at least) thirty-four weeks. The hospital I was in didn't have a Neonatal Intensive Care Unit (NICU), so if I had the baby before thirty-four weeks, I would need to be transferred to Brisbane. So, we had a goal: thirty-four weeks. And a plan: stay still.

The waiting game began. Paul was meant to be overseas doing his last round of shows – including a weekend in New York – but he cancelled to be with me. We didn't know when I was going to go into labour, but we knew when it did happen, it could be quick because of how short my cervix was. Paul didn't want to be on the other side of the world when things kicked off. We had waited so long for our baby, he wasn't going to miss the birth for anything.

Of course, it was still a tough call to cancel the shows. It really cut Paul up to let people down. We thought we'd planned his schedule perfectly around the due date, but we didn't expect this spanner in the works. It was a parenting lesson in the making: babies don't give a shit about your schedule. Our baby was large, and most definitely in charge.

In my room at the hospital, I was horizontal for a week. I felt okay. Yes, I was heavily pregnant and feeling the weight of that, but I was well. Most importantly, the baby was well too. However, I did feel a bit delirious. I kept drifting off into my own little world and couldn't stay focused. It was very unlike me. Luckily, I had some top-tier entertainment in Paul, Ellidy and Minnie, who charmed the nurses into giving her tubs of the hospital ice-cream and cans of lemonade. I also had two seasons of *Heartbreak High* (the new series, not the OG with Drazic), which I binge-watched with Paul on Netflix.

Most afternoons, Paul would pick Minnie up from kindy and bring her for a visit. I always heard her before I saw her. She would run down the corridor squealing, 'Coco, Coco, I miss Coco.' She loved cuddling my belly, but I'm not sure she knew what it meant.

After a week on my best behaviour, I was given a day pass to leave the hospital for my Australian baby shower, which Laura and Ellidy had organised. Before I was given the all-clear to attend, the nurses on my ward offered to let us have the shower in the hospital. 'You do not want sixty of my friends wreaking havoc in here,' I joked. 'Plus, I don't know if there's enough room for the girls' margarita station . . .'

It felt like a luxury to be going outside after being relegated to my hospital bed for a week. The girls knew I had to take it easy and not move around too much. When I arrived, I was a little overwhelmed by how many people were there and how much love was in the room.

I felt a bit like royalty sitting in the middle of the room, having people bring me things to eat and drink. All I could do was sit. And eat. The catering was off the hook. I ate so many meatballs, mini cheeseburgers, pastries and zucchini flowers. Naturally, lunch was followed by cake, which was a huge hit. I hate the word 'moist', but this cake was so ridiculously moist. I still think about it.

Apart from the food, one of my favourite moments from the day was the mother's blessing by my friend Faye. Everyone at the shower gave me a bead with a wish for my birth. Most people brought beautiful rose quartz and crystal beads; Ellidy brought a dog bead that looked like Scooby-Doo. Classic Ell.

Faye took all the beads and threaded them onto string so I could wear them as a necklace – or clutch them like pearls – during my birth, knowing I had the strength and support of my friends with me.

It was such a wondrous experience. I remember how much I struggled seeing other people's baby showers when I was aching to be pregnant, so I didn't take it for granted for a second. I was so grateful to Laura and Ell for organising, and Mon for hosting. And to all my friends for coming. So much so, I spent a little too long on my goodbyes and missed my 'curfew'.

In the car on the way 'home', the hospital called to see where I was. Not to worry! I was on my way back – and I was bringing cake. I took the leftover cake back to my ward for the nurses and staff, and it didn't last the night. It was the talk of the hospital. Hot tip: nurses really love cake.

I was in the good books with the nurses, and back on bed rest. Getting through my baby shower without going into labour felt like an achievement. *Hang in there, little baby,* I thought as I rubbed my belly.

I had a sinking feeling the baby would arrive on Saturday, 4 May 2024. For months, Paul had been working on launching his own festival – Out 2 Lunch – and the gig was scheduled for that day. He'd poured his heart and soul into the event, and it was set to be the biggest beach party in Coolangatta history, with a record-breaking 30,000 attendees.

If the baby had Paul's trickster sense of humour, I thought for sure it would make its debut appearance during his set time, which was between 7 and 9 pm. I had visions of Paul stepping off the stage and having to rush straight back to the hospital to cut the umbilical cord.

I didn't make it to Paul's set at Coolangatta, but the team organised a live stream so I could watch my love in action. It was my first time seeing his new show and I was in absolute awe. Paul had just released a remixed J.Lo track, 'Waiting for Tonight', and he was frothing to play it live. In the background, waves crashed on the beach and the sun set below the horizon, bathing everyone in golden light. On the stage, the smile on Paul's face was golden too. And he had every reason to smile; Out 2 Lunch was his vision, and he'd made it a reality.

Paul called me straight after his set. 'That was the best show I've ever played,' he said. 'I've never experienced that energy.'

Ell, who'd been in the crowd, said the exact same thing. 'That's my best friend, that's my best friend,' she kept saying to anyone who would listen. The vibrations from the crowd were electric; they roared for Paul. The sea of 30,000 people was united by the music. What a rush. Ell cried with pride for her Brother Fish.

I was sad to have missed the show, as you would expect, but I was so pleased that the sonographer had spotted my shortened cervix when they did. Can you imagine if I'd been bouncing around in a crowd of 30,000 people, not knowing I was at the stage directly before labour!? My waters would have broken for sure.

At the festival, a few people asked Ell where I was. She played dumb and said I was probably up in the VIP section or something. I hadn't announced publicly that I was in hospital – I didn't want people to think I was in labour, so we were keeping the bed rest on the downlow.

Back in my hospital bed the following week, Ell and I recorded an episode of *Darling, Shine!*, to be released a couple of weeks later. That's when I gave the update: 'As it stands, baby is comfortable here, and the baby's calling the shots.'

For once in my life, I was happy for someone else to take charge.

Before their arrival, I wrote a letter to my baby in my pregnancy book.

Dear Baby,

We are so close to meeting you, my heart swells with joy and excitement at the thought of finally holding you in my arms. Our journey to you has been filled with many ups and downs, but every moment has been worth it.

For the past four years, your arrival has been the dream that kept me going. There were times that the path seemed too difficult, and the hope of meeting you felt like a distant star. But through it all, we never gave up!

Every tear shed, every doctor visit, every prayer whispered was a step closer to you. Your dad and I have grown so much through this journey. We've learned about resilience, the power of hope and the depth of unconditional love.

As your due date approaches, I find myself dreaming of what you will look like, the sound of your first cry, the feeling of your tiny fingers wrapped around mine. I promise to cherish every moment with you, from the sleepless nights to your first steps and every second in between.

You are our miracle, our rainbow after the storm, and we cannot wait to show you just how much you are loved. So deeply loved by so many; your grandparents, aunties, uncles, and friends waiting patiently to shower you with love and affection.

We will be there to guide and support you and celebrate with you every step of the way. We promise to provide you with a home filled with love, laughter and kindness. Thank you for choosing us to be your parents. You are our greatest gift, and we are so blessed to have you. We can't wait to meet you and begin this incredible journey together as a family.

Love, Mum xx

I was experiencing 'lightning crotch' when I wrote the letter. It genuinely felt like I'd been given an electric shock down there. The baby's head was engaged and pinching on nerves, which sent painful currents through my pelvic area – hence the name. The sparks didn't scare me, they excited me. I had dreamed of giving birth for so long, and I knew my dreams were going to come true sooner rather than later.

I wrote a birth plan. Of course I did. The plan was to have a dark room with fairy lights, a diffuser with lavender oil, a push playlist, an exercise ball, and time in the bath.

Paul was my birth partner, with Ellidy as back-up support. I knew I wanted – and needed – Ell in the delivery room with me, but I was worried about asking her to be there. I didn't want to be insensitive. I didn't want Ell to see me and Paul having our baby and remember that she didn't have Chumpy at Minnie's birth. When I worked up the courage to ask her though, Ell was so happy. 'This is the biggest honour,' she said.

Ell's first piece of advice to me was to throw the birth plan out the window. 'Nothing goes to plan, sis, there's no point having a plan,' she said, reminding me of how she'd wanted to have a water birth with Minnie, but was unable to because she didn't fit in the bath at the hospital.

After two weeks on bed rest, I was pretty over it. I had to put my phone on do-not-disturb mode because so many people were checking in on me, but I simply didn't have an update to give them. It was business as usual: waiting, waiting, waiting. Knowing so many people were playing the waiting game too made me feel anxious. Everyone wanted news, but I didn't have any to share.

Being in the hospital started to feel like overkill. I had made it past the thirty-four-week mark, and I really wanted to go home. I spoke to the doctors – and even googled 'can a hospital legally stop you from leaving?' – and pleaded my case. I promised I would stay still and horizontal at home, and I was given the okay on those conditions.

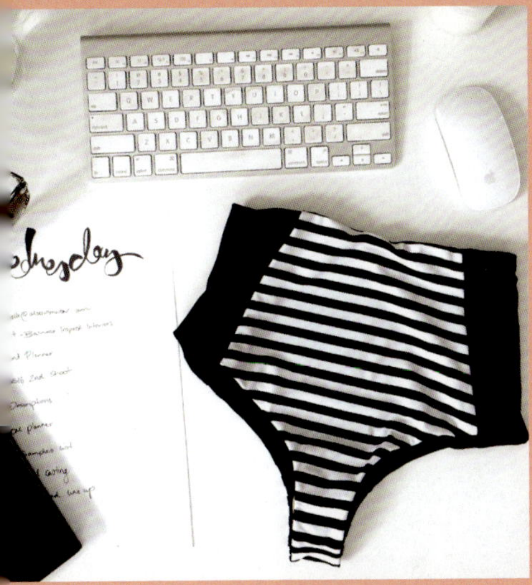

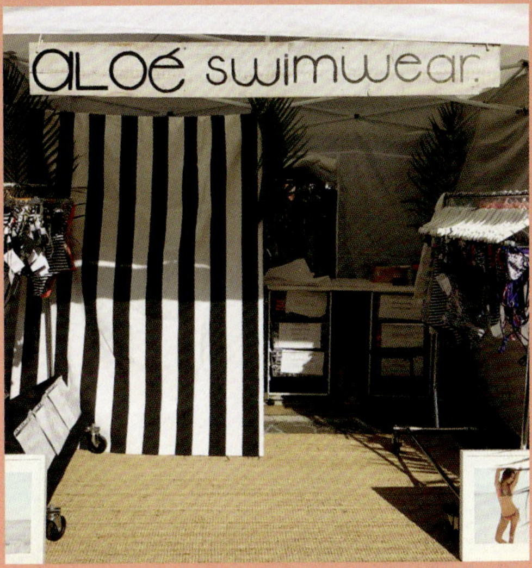
aLOé swimwear

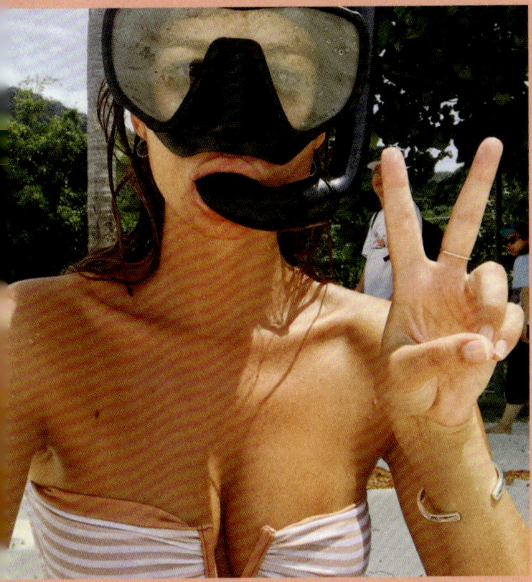

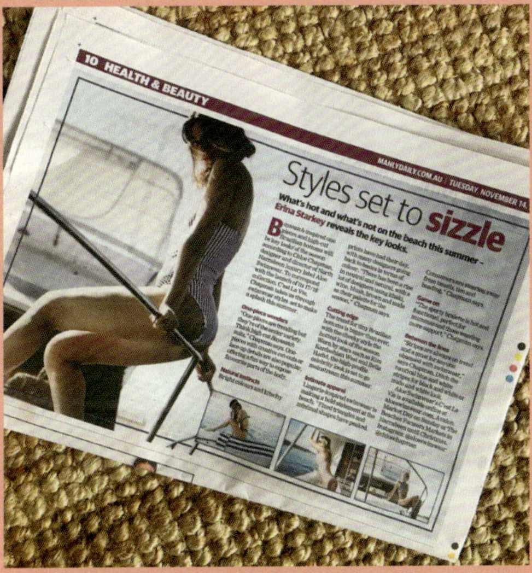
10 HEALTH & BEAUTY
Styles set to sizzle
What's hot and what's not on the beach this summer – Erina Starkey reveals the key looks.

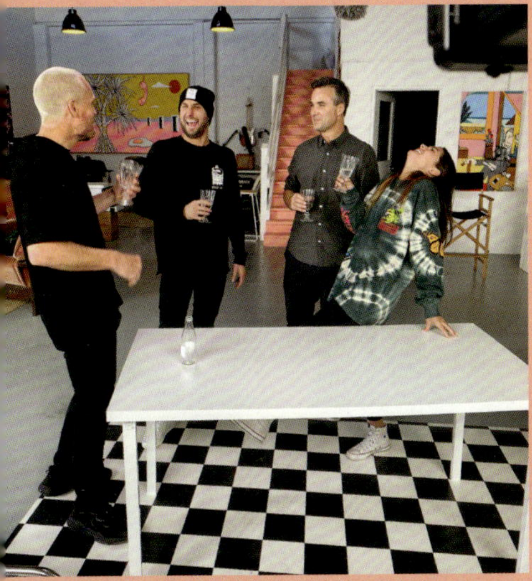

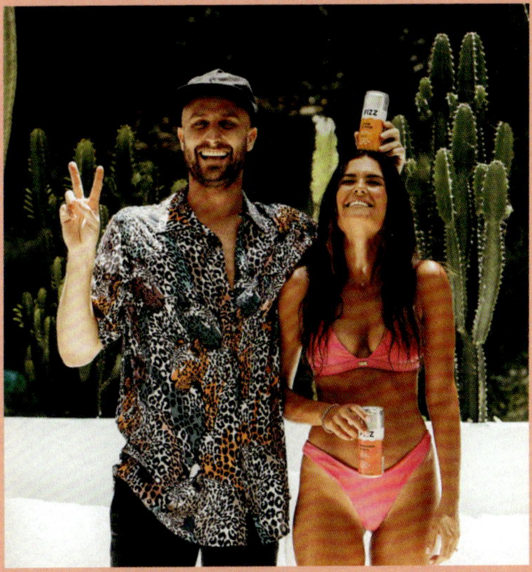

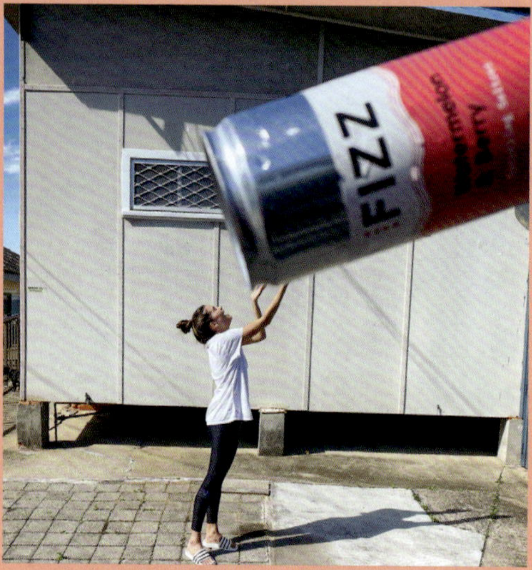
FIZZ

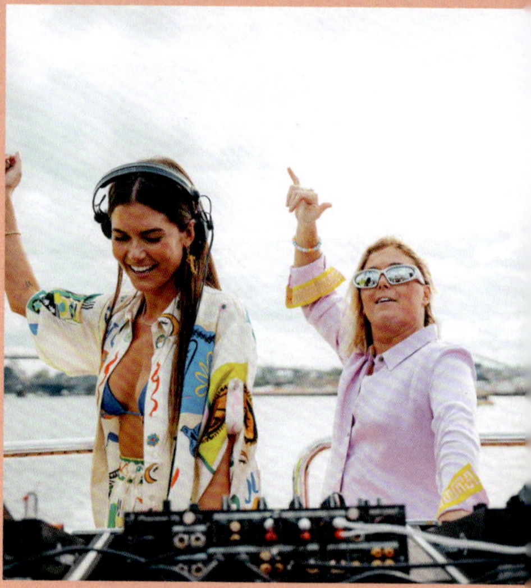

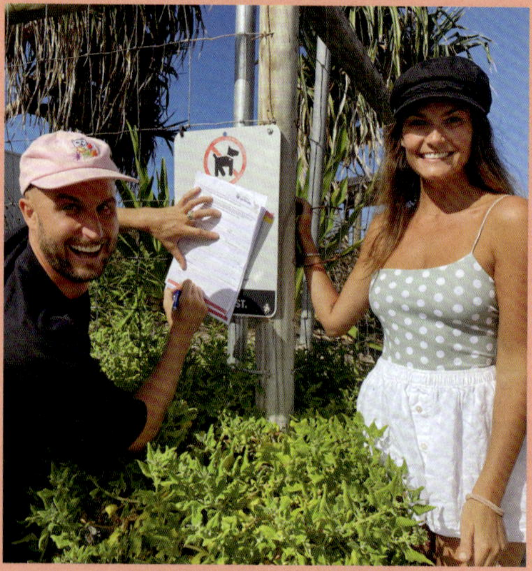

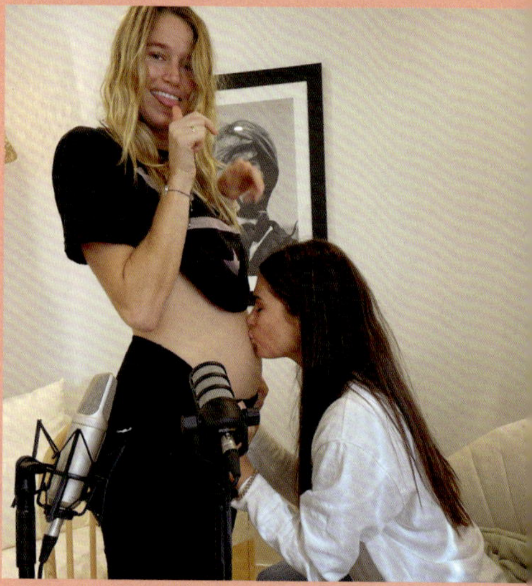

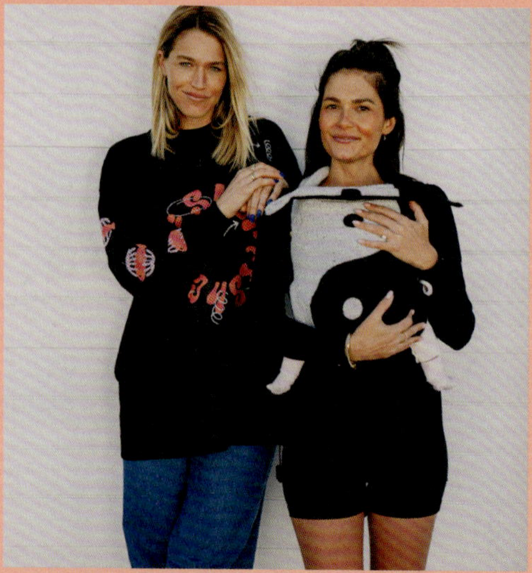

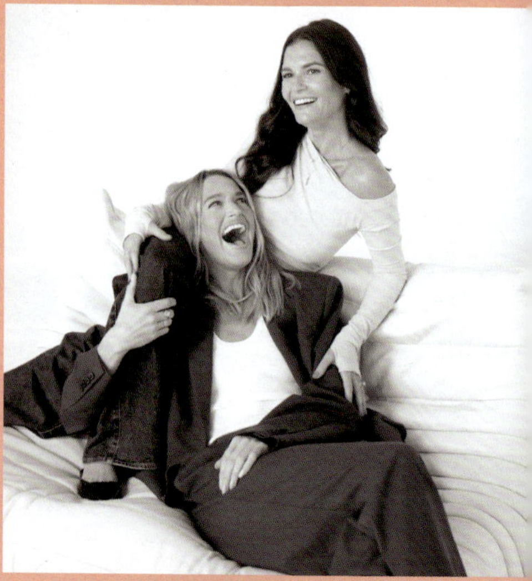

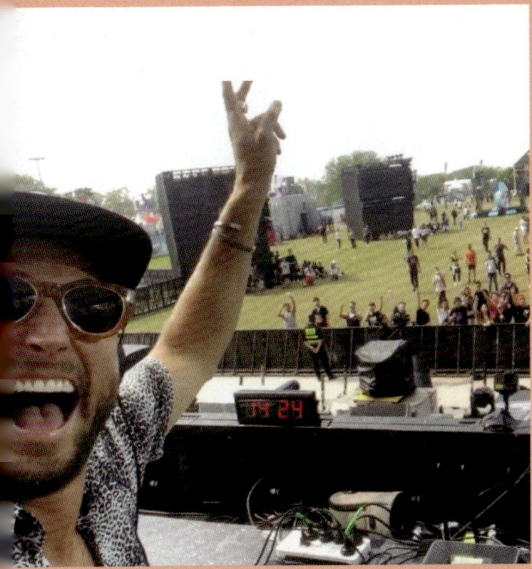

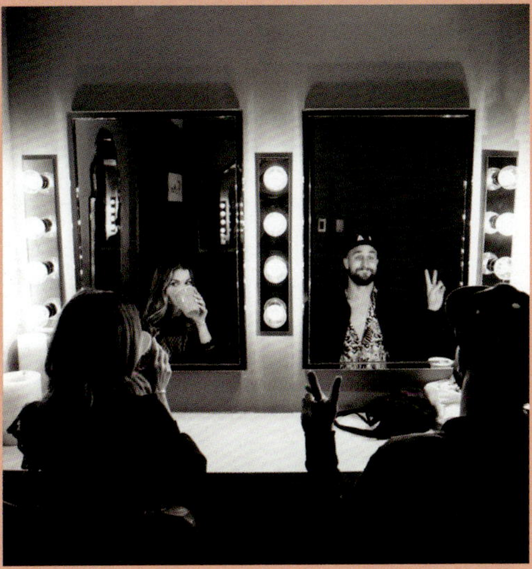

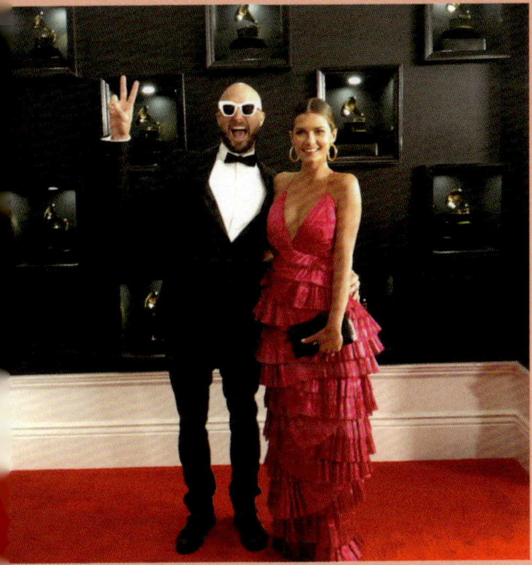

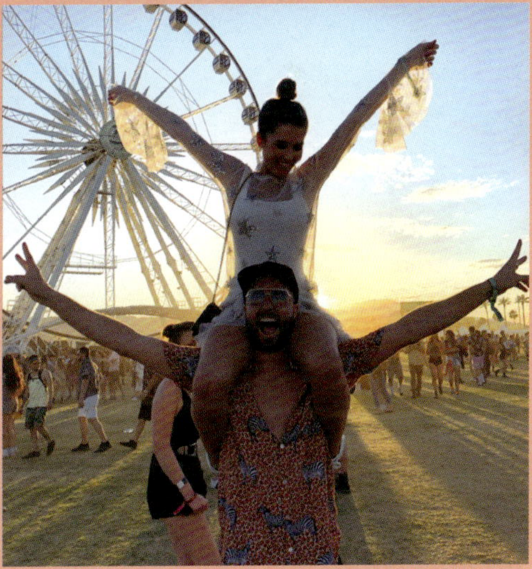

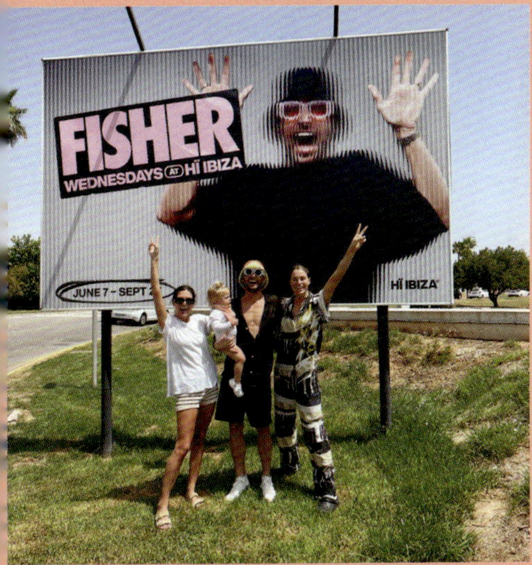
FISHER
WEDNESDAYS AT HÏ IBIZA
JUNE 7 – SEPT
HÏ IBIZA

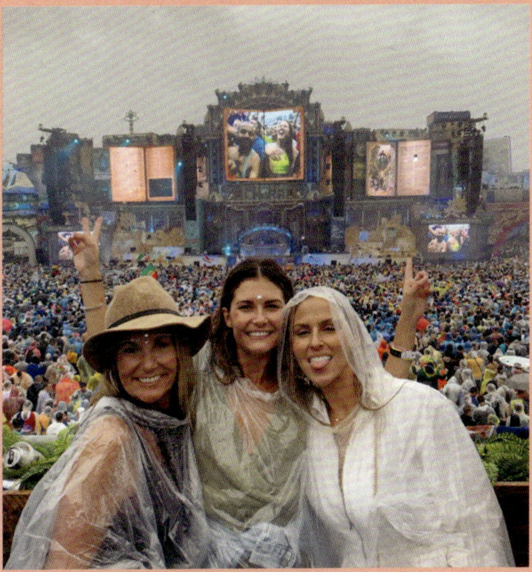

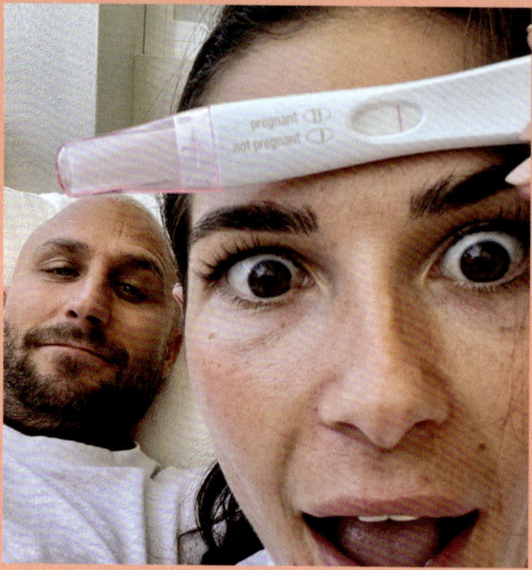
pregnant
not pregnant

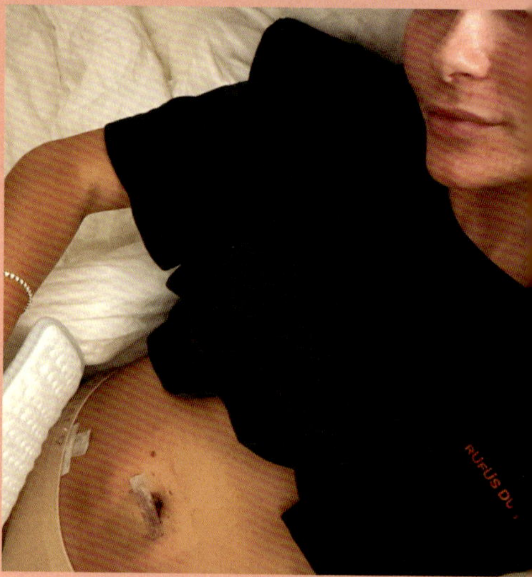

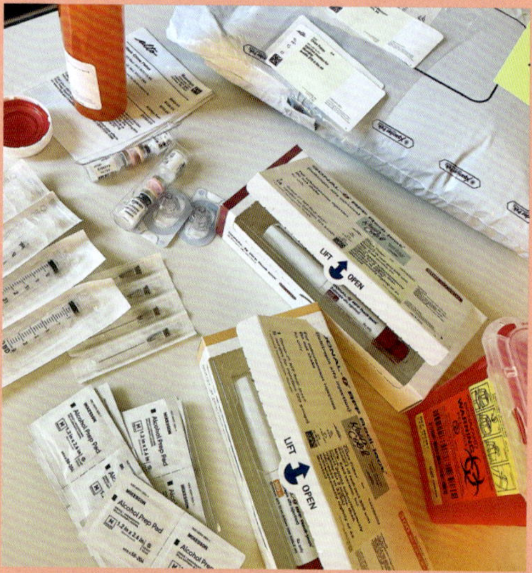
LIFT
OPEN
Alcohol Prep Pad

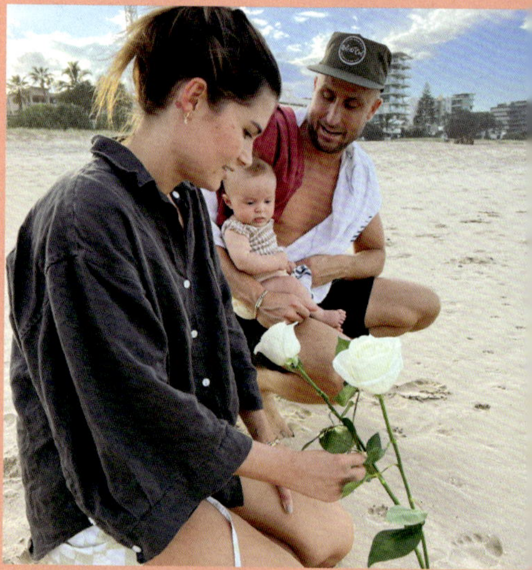

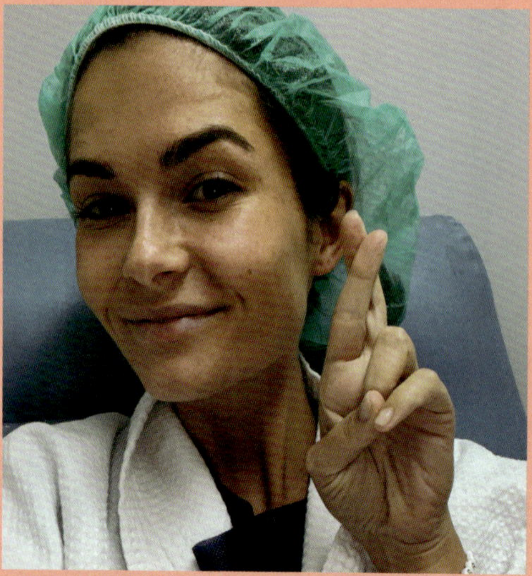

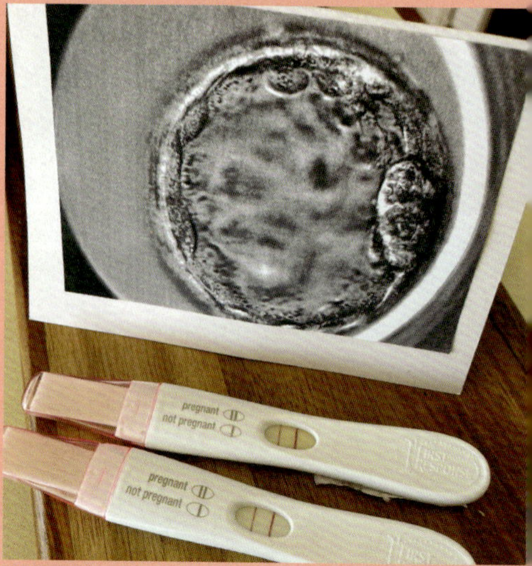
pregnant
not pregnant
pregnant
not pregnant

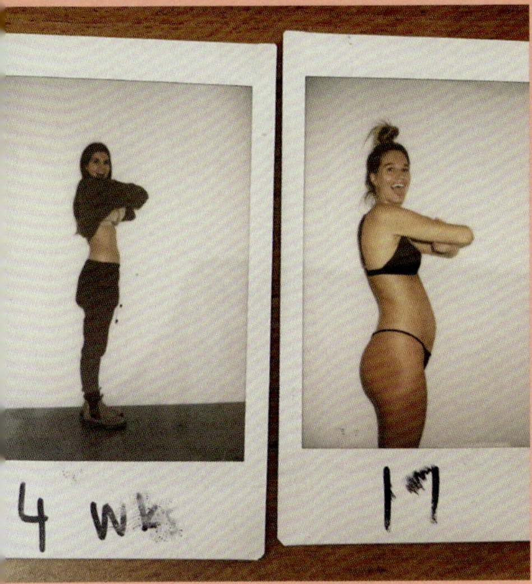
4 wk
17

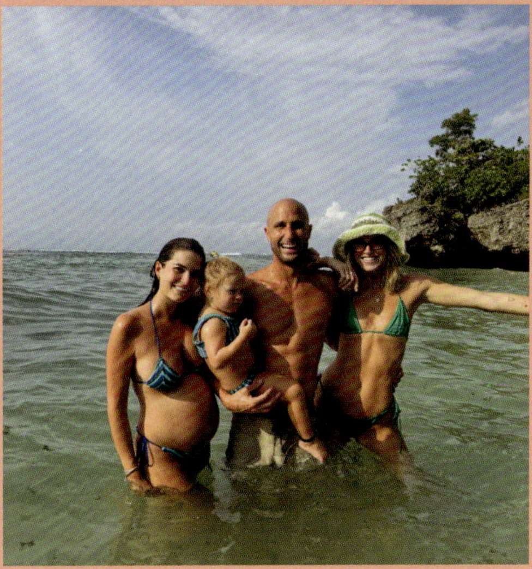

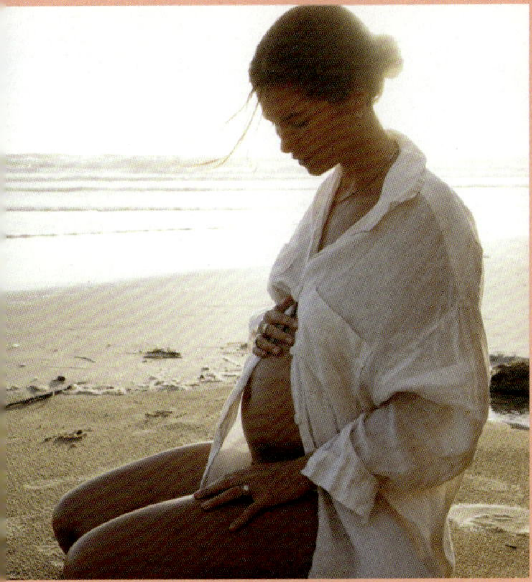

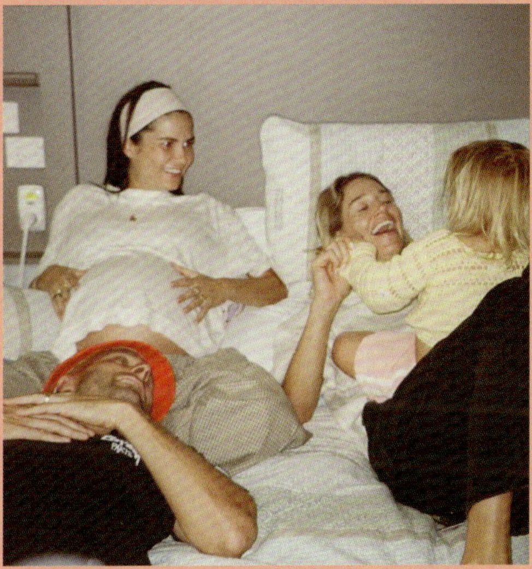

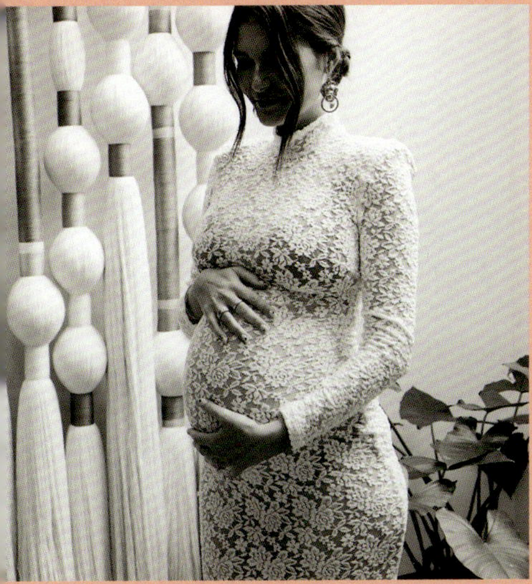

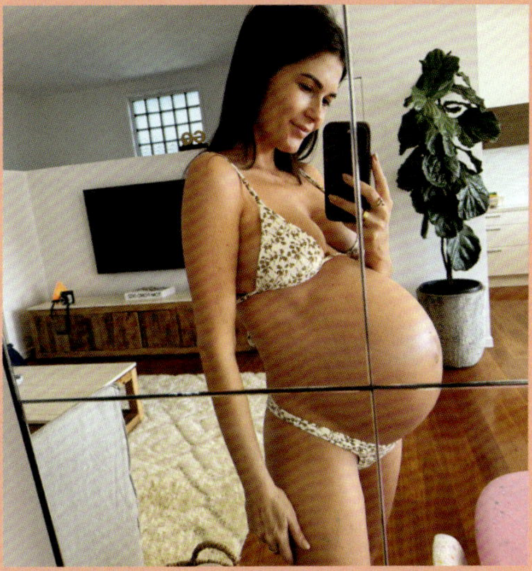

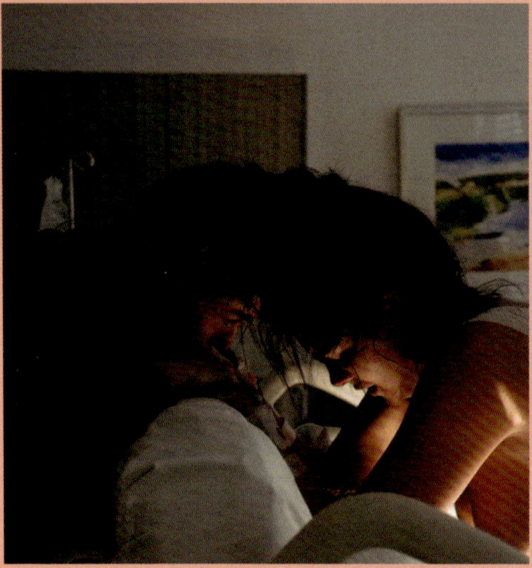
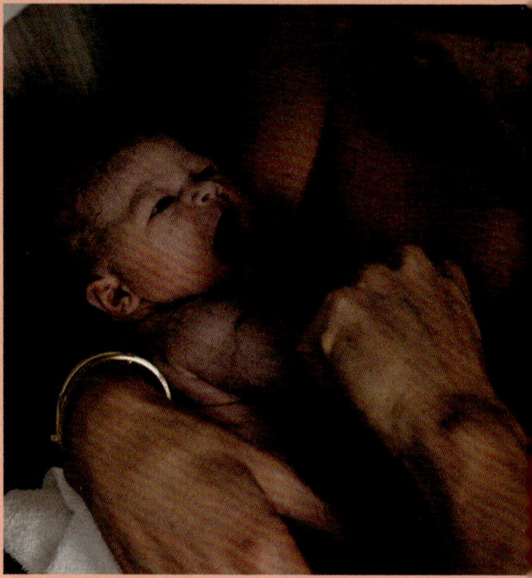
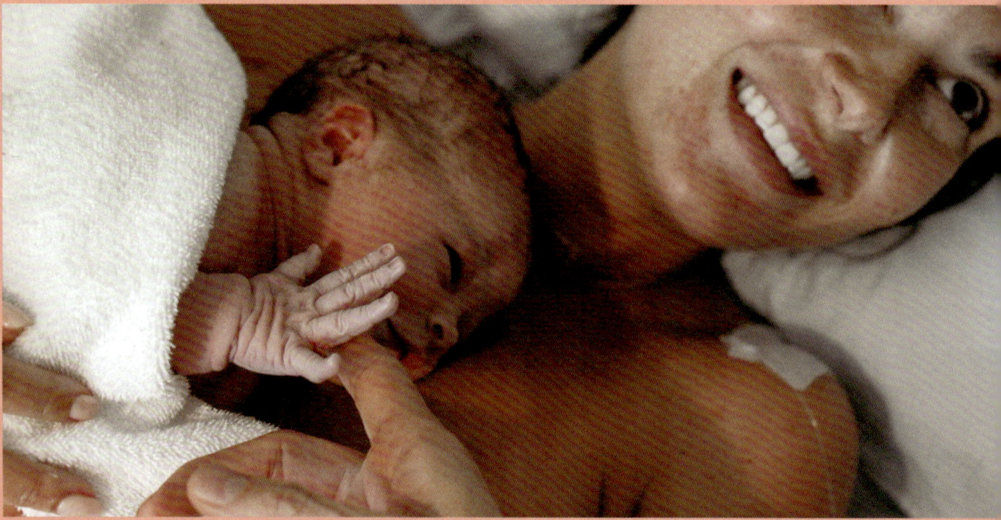
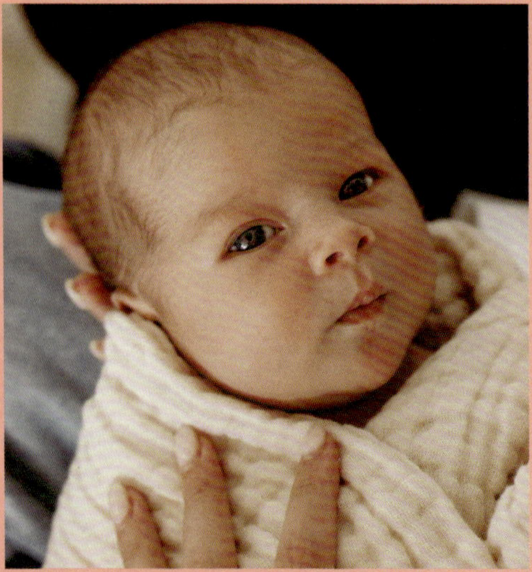
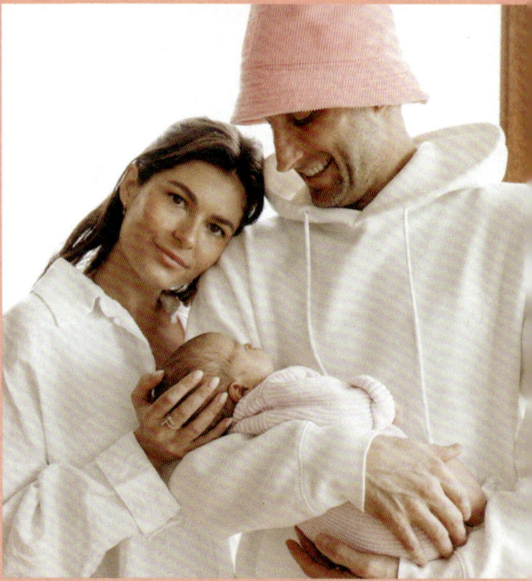

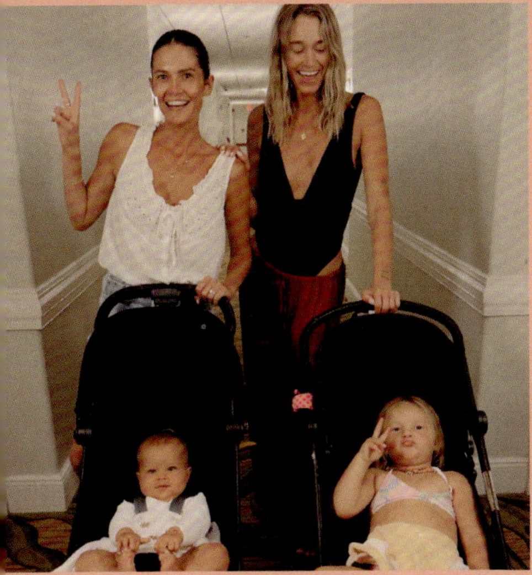

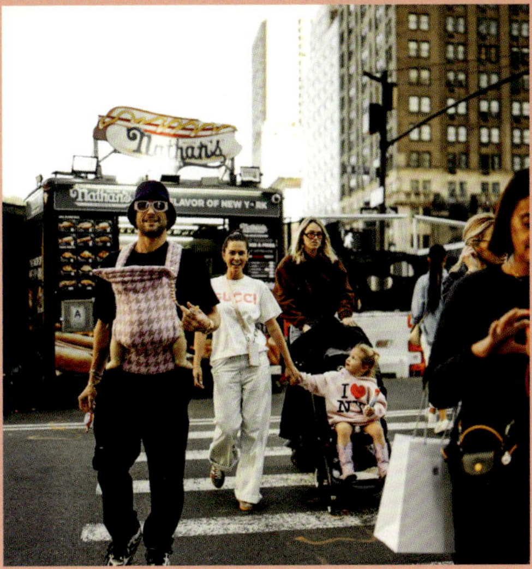
Nathan's

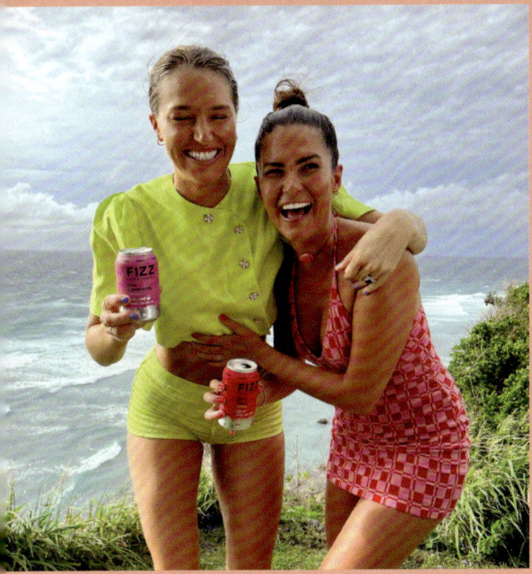
FIZZ

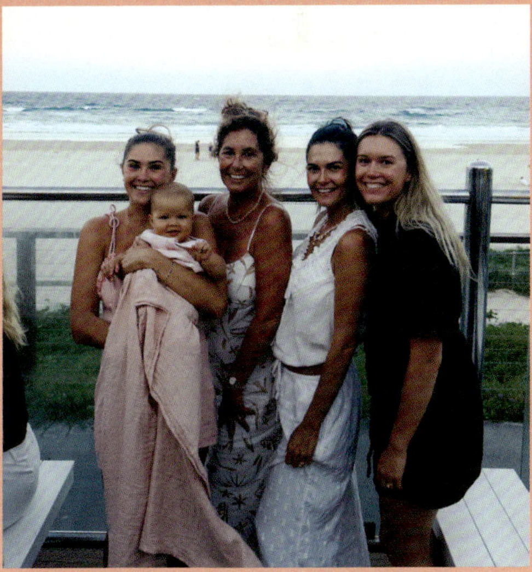

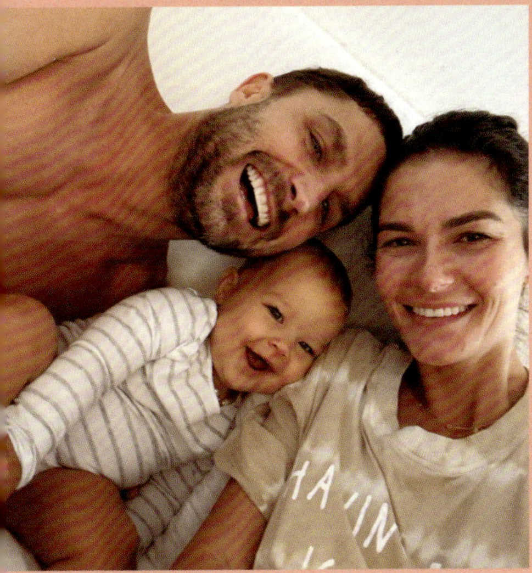

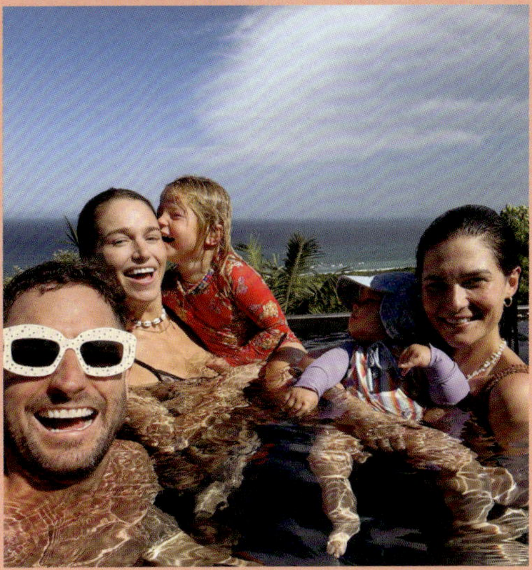

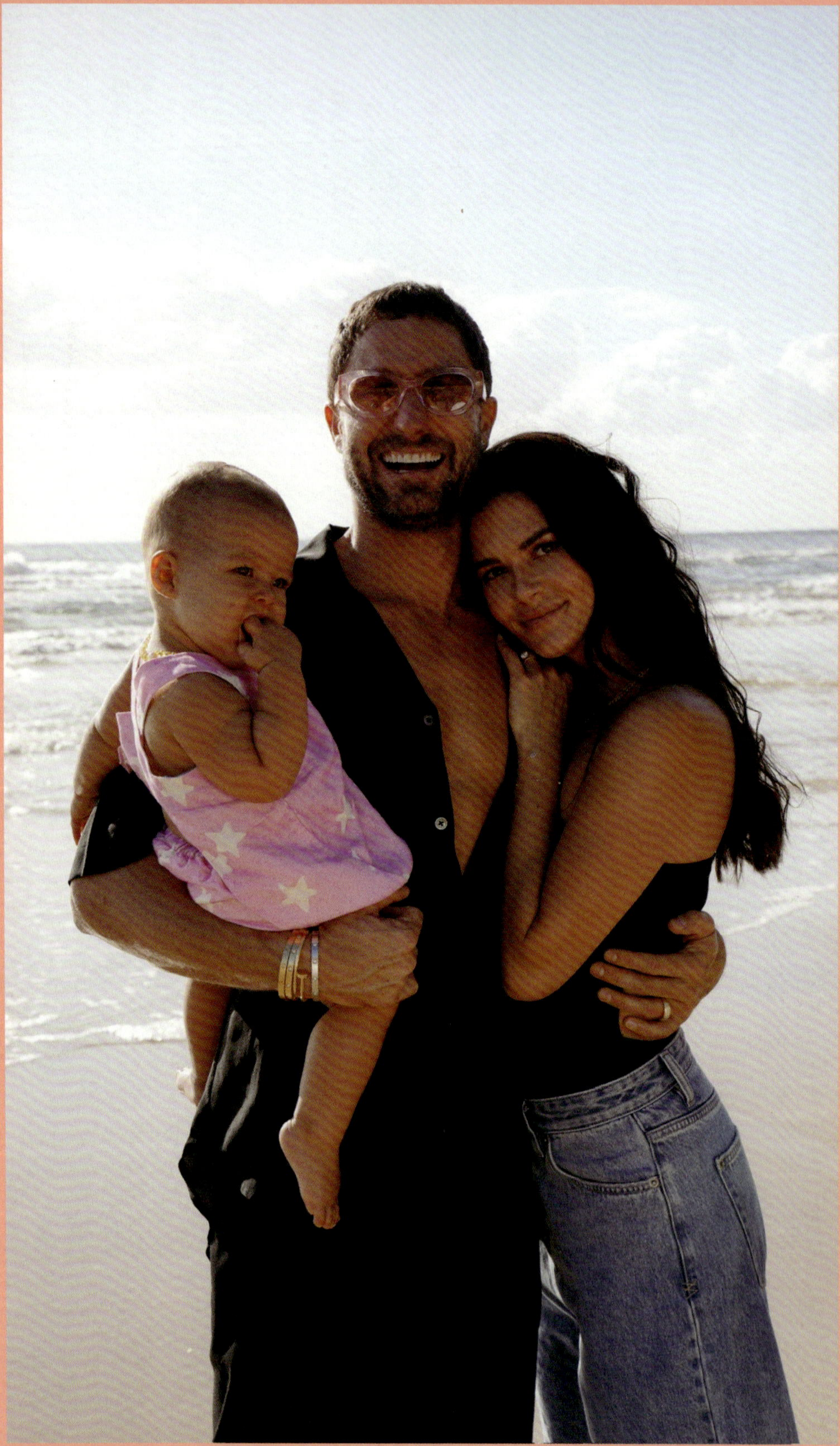

Back in our home, I went straight into nesting mode. I was able to finish getting the nursery ready and packed my hospital bag – with help from my mum, who'd come up to the Goldy for the impending birth. Paul risked it and went away for a few days to do some final shows before the arrival of our baby. While he was away, Ell, Minnie and Rummi came to stay with me. Rummi didn't leave my side, which was unusual for her. It was like she was guarding me and my belly. I was grateful for the protection.

It had been months since I'd seen my groin. I booked an appointment at a shopping centre beauty salon to get my bikini area waxed in anticipation for the birth. As I was laying on the bed with my legs spread, I told the beauty therapist how excited I was about giving birth. 'I don't know why,' she replied. 'It's the worst thing you'll ever go through. I can't even begin to describe the pain to you. It's fucked.'

As she spoke, she pulled a wax strip off with such force that it flew out of her hand and stuck to the wall behind her. It was hilarious; we both cracked up. The laughter almost drowned out her warning. Almost.

The essentials

What to pack in your hospital bag for the maternity ward

THE USUAL SUSPECTS

- Your birth plan or requests for people present in your birthing suite
- Oversized pair of PJs, tees and comfy pants
- Maternity bras and crops without underwire
- Loose full-brief underwear
- A pair of slippers
- Hydration sachets
- Depending on the size of the baby, a handful of size 00000 zip onesies
- Cloth for spew and nappies
- Extra-absorbent maxi pads (the hospital will provide them, but you might want to use your favourite brand instead).

THE GAME CHANGERS

- A water bottle with a *bendy straw*! My Hydro Flask bottle was a total lifesaver during labour.
- Some lanolin for your lips (also great for cracked or sensitive nipples).
- A headband for labour to keep your hair out of your face.
- A push playlist. Paul's US agent, Cody, made me a playlist featuring classics like 'Ring of Fire', 'The Final Countdown'

and 'Always Be My Baby', which you can find on Spotify if you search 'Chloe's Push Playlist'. I also made a calm back-up playlist for the moments when Cody's was too intense; search 'Birth Suite by Chloe' to hear this one.

- Something sentimental. I had a crystal chain, which was made by collecting the beads from my baby shower. I genuinely felt the energy and love from my friends having that visible in the room with me.
- Battery-powered fairy lights.
- A diffuser and sound machine to set the mood. I loved having lavender oil diffused in my room.
- Frida Mom Labour and Post Partum Recovery Kit (check them out online, this kit was the GOAT for me). The disposable pants were a godsend! Better than any other adult nappies I came across.
- Extra-long phone charger.
- Your favourite pillow and an extra pillowslip.

Fifteen

WORTH THE WAIT

In all the pregnancy journals I bought and owned before 2024, I never got to write a birth story. That changed in June. My pen was primed to document every moment of my labour.

We were ready. We knew the baby could come at any time. Paul was home from his shows, and the first thing he did when he got back was put a garbage bag down on the passenger seat of our car so I wouldn't stain the leather with bodily fluids when I went into labour. Ever the clean freak.

I had been feeling so confident about giving birth. My energy-charged beads were in my hospital bag, and I felt ready, strong and prepared. Then the Braxton Hicks started. The 'practice contractions', which happen when the uterine muscle relaxes ahead of birth, were sharp and sore. The pain jolted me, and I began to feel nervous about my baby's impending birth. For my entire life – even during the agony of the previous five years – I'd had an unshakeable belief that I would have a baby. Suddenly I doubted I could do it. I didn't want to be afraid, but I was.

I chatted to Ell on a podcast episode about how my Braxton Hicks contractions had rattled me, and her advice didn't exactly help. 'Hang on doll, those period pains that you're getting now are fuck all compared to what you're about to endure,' she said. 'Get the epi[dural] though, you'll be right!'

I started to cross things off my birth plan. I didn't see how holding onto a labour comb would help me with the agony. I no longer cared about getting my placenta encapsulated into tablets or having a salt lamp beside me. All I wanted was to get through the pain and deliver a healthy baby.

The things I cared about were the basics. I wanted Paul to be there to grab the baby when it arrived and announce whether it was a boy or girl. I wanted to delay the cord clamping for as long as possible for the health benefits (increased blood volume, iron stores and improved circulation) for the baby. And I wanted my friend Karina, who is a brilliant photographer, to capture the baby's first moments Earthside.

A silver lining to having such a long fertility journey was that I got to know the doctors, nurses, midwives and hospital staff really well. After spending a fortnight on the maternity ward on bed rest, I knew how things worked – and, most importantly, how capable everyone was. The team delivered babies every single day; it was their bread and butter. I trusted them implicitly and knew they wouldn't do anything that went against my wishes. I felt like I was in safe hands.

On 19 June, I wrote one word on the Thirty-Nine Weeks page in my pregnancy journal: '*INDUCED*!' It was written in capitals with an exclamation mark and an underline.

After (impatiently) waiting to go into labour, the call was made for me to have an induction. Because I wanted to try to have a vaginal birth and because the baby was so big, I chose to be induced. I was open to having a C-section if it was necessary, but I wanted to try this first.

I was set to be admitted to hospital at 3 pm on 19 June to begin the process. Paul and I started the day by watching the sunrise over the beach. He rubbed my belly and I talked to the baby. It was perfect. At lunch, we met Ellidy and Minnie, and Laura and her boyfriend Jake, at our favourite restaurant, Pipi's. We went straight from the restaurant to the hospital. It felt like we were driving toward our destiny.

At the hospital that afternoon, Paul filmed a video of me, capturing the start of our emotional roller-coaster. I was sobbing as he spoke. 'You're about to be a mum,' he said. 'We've been waiting for this for a while. How special. It's going to be the best day of our lives.'

'Hello mate,' he said to my belly. 'It's time to meet your parents, time to be a Fisher.'

At 5 pm I was given a dose of Prostin gel, which was inserted into my vagina to help soften and dilate the neck of the womb to bring on labour. Paul and I ate dinner in my hospital room – our last meal as just the two of us – and soaked up the time together.

Throughout the night, we took more videos and photos for prosperity; the moments before our life would change forever. In all the images, Paul was wearing one of his trademark bucket hats. We knew people would wonder why on earth he had a hat on inside, at night. The truth was, Paul had got a hair transplant a month earlier. It was something he'd been considering doing for three years, and he'd finally gone in and had the procedure done at a Brisbane clinic. By the time I was induced, Paul had stubble growing on his head – the transplant had worked! – and it looked really good.

We knew if we shared photos of him from the hospital without a hat on, everyone would focus on his miraculous new hairdo. So, Paul chucked on a hat, even though some people might think he was a wanker for doing so. Paul wanted the moment to be about me and our baby, not his hairline.

By 10 pm, when we did the second dose of Prostin, I was two to three centimetres dilated. I started having small, slow contractions almost immediately. I'd been having Braxton Hicks in the weeks leading up to this, and I didn't know if I would be able to tell the difference between them and actual contractions. Everyone told me not to worry, I would definitely know when I was having a real contraction. They were right.

The contractions hit, and they hit hard. I started to time them on an app. I was lying on one bed in the room and Paul was on another. We didn't speak; I focused on my breathing, and Paul focused on me. When a contraction took hold, I repeated the same phrase over and over: 'It's one step closer to meeting my baby, one step closer, one step closer.'

When a nurse came to check on me and I showed her the contraction timings on the app, she said, 'Oh yeah, we're on here.'

At midnight, one of my midwives, Jasmine, ran a bath for me in the birthing suite. Paul turned on our fairy lights and I sank into the water. 'For me, that moment was so beautiful,' Paul said later. 'Chloe was in the bath, and in the zone. It was quiet and calm.'

The connection I felt with Paul in those moments was magical. I had never felt closer to him – or more in love with him. It was almost euphoric. I captured the memory in my mind because I knew I would want to revisit it over and over again.

As beautiful as it was, it was equally brutal. I went from the bath to the bed, and from the bed to the bath. The pain was white-hot. It burned. By 3 am, I needed pain relief. I was given a shot of pethidine, which took the edge off for an hour and a half. At that point, I requested an epidural. I was told I had to wait 45 minutes for the anaesthetist to arrive, and that was the longest 45 minutes of my life. I've never wanted a needle more.

At 5 am, I was finally given the epidural. When the anaesthetist finished, he asked Paul for a photo. He was a fan. It was a classic. While Paul was taking selfies, I messaged my other midwife, Lisa, who came in early for her shift and didn't leave my side. Lisa used to work at Dr Ong's fertility clinic and had held my hands through many tough appointments. Another midwife was Clare, who I'd followed on Instagram when I found out I was pregnant this time around and who looked after me during my bed rest stay in hospital. I was so thankful to have them both there.

Lisa broke my waters. It was a bit anticlimactic, to be honest. There wasn't an almighty rush of water, which we'd been expecting because I was carrying so much fluid.

The energy shifted as the sun began to rise on 20 June. The night had been so dream-like, but after the epidural, it felt like go time. I had been feeling pretty out of it, but the pain relief brought me back to life. Paul and I high-fived, I brushed my teeth, combed my hair, giggled and put my push playlist on. 'My Girl' by The Temptations was playing, Lisa was dancing, I was fist-pumping and Paul was crying on the phone to Brett in the States. It was such a vibe.

I was too nauseous to eat, but I was slowly chewing on some energy gummies my brother had given me. Cooper had run a hundred-kilometre marathon a few months earlier and had some of the lollies left over. He thought they might help me during birth, which was a different kind of marathon. I was certainly drinking like I was running. The hospital felt like the Sahara Desert. I was so thirsty and dry. I was constantly sipping water and asking Paul to put lip gloss on my lips.

I called my mum to update her on the progress, and she was at Sydney airport waiting to board a flight to the Gold Coast. It was 6.30 am and she was having a Bloody Mary. I had to cut the call short after she told me that. The words 'Bloody Mary' made me physically ill. So much so, I filled two vomit bags. I don't know if I'll ever be able to drink a Bloody Mary again.

After a few hours, the epidural started to wear off, and I asked the anaesthetist for a top-up. The drugs did the job – I was completely numb from the waist down – but it was such a strange feeling. I felt disconnected from my body.

My midwives told me I was getting close. I messaged Ellidy and Karina and asked them to get to the hospital asap. I genuinely thought I was moments away from giving birth and I was worried they would miss it. They needn't have rushed; I hadn't even started pushing yet. I was nowhere near 'close'.

When Ell was saying goodbye to Minnie that morning, she told her there was a surprise coming for her later. 'You're getting a baby brother or sister this afternoon,' Ell said.

I was ten centimetres dilated when Ellidy and Karina arrived at the hospital at around 10 am. By that point I had been in hospital for nineteen hours, and having contractions for twelve. I was excited, and relieved to see the girls. Ell was in full Energiser bunny mode, cheekily taking hits on the gas (which was only pumping out oxygen) and running amok. The energy in the room was high.

After 11 am, Lisa told me to start pushing. I knew I had to push from my bum, but I couldn't physically do it. My lower half was entirely numb. I tried and I tried, but I couldn't get my muscles to do what I wanted. It was frustrating and disorienting. We made the decision to lower the pain relief I was getting from the epidural so I could get some feeling back. To go from totally numb to full-force pain was wild.

The contractions got closer together, the pain got more intense and the self-doubt got louder. After pushing for what felt like hours, my midwives swore I was 'so close'. They put a mirror between my legs to show me, and I could tell I had so much further to go. I lost hope. I felt so disheartened.

I screamed at Paul – who was being so amazing and supportive – and let him have it. 'I am one and done! If you think I'm having another baby, you're tripping, that ain't happening. I can never go through this again,' I said.

The energy in the room was too high. There was too much noise. I needed to lower the vibrations and the noise. The midwives understood the assignment and asked Ellidy and Karina to go and grab some morning tea from the common area. They happily obliged.

In the hospital bed, every move was excruciating. I rolled over onto my side and gripped onto the bars of the bed with both hands. Paul was beside the bed, kneeling so he was at eye-level with me. His face was full of concern. Mine was scrunched with pain. I couldn't handle it. I started vomiting. Paul started crying and patting my back.

I had a holy-shit moment. *I can't do this,* I thought. *I think I'm going to die. I need to make this pain stop.*

I racked my brain for ways to stop the pain, but I realised the only way it would stop was if I birthed the baby. I reminded myself that women give birth every day, that our bodies are built for it, that I was built for it. That knowledge didn't really help at the time.

I swear no-one explicitly told me just how fucked birth is, except for the beauty therapist who did my bikini wax before I was induced. Ellidy says she tried to, but I mustn't have comprehended what she was saying. I think because everyone knew how desperate I was to have a baby, no-one wanted to be brutally honest about labour. They didn't want to trash talk the thing I wanted most in the world. Even if someone had spelled it out for me, I don't think you can fully understand how hectic birth is until you've experienced it.

When Ell came back from morning tea, she was more serious and focused. Or maybe I was more desperate, and she could see how much I was struggling. She knew exactly where I was – in a deep hole of despair. She had been there too. And she'd gotten out of it.

Ell got right in my face and started pushing with me. She made some animalistic noises, encouraging me to do the same. 'Be an animal,' she urged me. 'Scream like an animal.'

Clare says ours was the loudest delivery room she's ever been in. The noise wasn't coming from me, though. 'You were so serene, Chloe,' Clare told me later. 'You really went within and did what needed to be done. Your focus was next-level.'

'You can do this Chloe,' the room – Paul, Ellidy, Lisa and Clare – told me.

I didn't know if I could. I was pushing with all my might, and the baby's head was showing, but as soon as I stopped, the head would go back inside me. I couldn't get the baby those extra few millimetres out. I found out later that the baby's head was bouncing off my pelvis.

After fifteen hours of labour, I begged to be taken to surgery for a C-section. I was done. The pain had won. I had nothing left to give. When my obstetrician came in after midday, he offered to do a forceps delivery with an episiotomy. 'Yes, absolutely, just get this baby out of me,' I agreed.

The epidural was pumped back up and I was given more gas. Paul held one of my legs and the doctor sat between them. The forceps were huge. The doctor asked Paul if he was okay; he must have looked like he was about to faint. I knew the feeling.

At my next contraction, the doctor inserted the forceps and got a grip on the baby's head. As I pushed, he pulled. The baby's head popped out and the room ignited with excitement. Paul was right there. His first thought was, *Jeez, this baby is so cute. They've been here before.*

The midwives encouraged me to reach down and feel the baby's head, which I did. *They're here, they're here,* I thought.

In the chaos of the moment, everyone forgot I still had to deliver the rest of the baby. The room went silent as I waited for my next contraction. The midwives had to keep feeling my belly to see when it hit because I was too numb from the epidural to know. I was given the episiotomy, where they cut from my vagina down toward my bum.

'Are you ready?' Lisa asked Paul, who was in position to deliver the baby.

'I'm ready! I'm ready!' he said.

Bon Iver played in the background as Paul pulled the baby out of me with some help from the doctor. He was afraid of dropping the baby because it was so slippery when it came out. As Paul brought the baby over to me, he said, 'It's a girl.'

I let out a noise I've never made before. It was something between a sigh, a roar, a sob and a squeal. I'll never forget that sound.

Paul gently placed our daughter on my chest, and I burst into guttural sobs. It was a moment I had envisioned for so long; a moment I had played over and over in my head when doubt crept in; a moment that gave me the hope to keep going. I lifted the baby up to check that she really was a girl. I couldn't believe she was real.

My baby girl was here, just like I always knew she would be. I felt it all: the weight of her tiny body on my chest, the sensation of her skin on my skin, the sound of her sweet little sigh. I felt whole.

'It's Bobbi girl,' Paul said. 'She's here.'

Bobbi Maree Fisher was born at 1.15 pm on 20 June 2024, weighing 3.49 kilograms. Her name was written in the front of my pregnancy journal. She had her dad's blue eyes and her mum's olive skin. She was the baby I had prayed for and the one I had envisioned.

Bobbi was destined to be.

It was always her.

Sixteen

AN UNTOLD STORY

THE ROOM WAS THICK WITH RELIEF. THERE WERE LITERAL cheers in the birthing suite when Bobbi was born. Paul and Ellidy were hugging, laughing and crying, and the midwives were smiling from ear to ear. I was overwhelmed with love for my daughter. Everything else – time, pain, the stitches I was being given – ceased to exist.

As I held Bobbi to my chest, she couldn't stop staring at Paul. I was so grateful for him. We'd done it. We were parents. I was a mum. To a baby girl!

I had convinced myself I was having a boy, because all of my other pregnancies were boys – and, also, because I really wanted a girl and didn't want to be disappointed. Bobbi was my wildest dream realised. She was absolutely perfect. The love I felt for her was limitless.

Birth was the most profound and transformative experience of my life. It felt like stepping into another world – Labour Land, it's real! It was a mix of pain and purpose, and it awoke a resilience from deep within me that I never knew existed. Little did I know, I was going to need that resilience . . .

I held Bobbi for less than an hour, staring into her eyes and kissing her forehead, before I started to feel strange. I was flat and spacey. I asked Paul to take Bobbi. My midwife took note. Later, she told me that when a mother passes her newborn baby to someone else by choice, it's a sign. Something wasn't right.

Ell made a passing comment about how pale I looked. She was leaving to give us some time together and to grab us all food. I requested a Happy Meal from McDonald's. She didn't mention how white I was again, for fear of offending me, but she was right. The colour had completely drained from my face. I was ghostly.

Lisa took my blood pressure. When the numbers came back, they were alarmingly low. The relief in the room turned to panic. Clare pressed the emergency button. She wasn't mucking around; she'd experienced a postpartum haemorrhage and suspected I was going through the same.

When Lisa checked out my vagina, she pulled clumps of blood out of me. Handful after handful. When she pushed down on my belly, even more blood gushed out. Paul described it as being like something out of a horror movie. He said I looked lifeless.

'Babe, are you okay?' he asked me.

I didn't reply. I just stared at him blankly. I wasn't there. I was gone.

In an instant, the happiest moment of my life became the scariest. It all happened so fast. Nurses came from everywhere. They laid me down flat in the bed and pushed me out the door, heading straight for the ER. One of the nurses paused. 'Paul, you should give Chloe a kiss,' she said. He came over with Bobbi and kissed my forehead.

As quickly as the nurses had descended on the room – like an F1 pit crew – they wheeled me out of it. Lisa held my hand as I was rushed down the corridor to the emergency elevator. I remember feeling like I was drifting off. I knew I wasn't hooked up to any machines or pain relief, so that wasn't the reason I was slipping away. *Is this what dying feels like?* I wondered. *Am I dying?*

Paul was wondering the same thing. He had been left alone, holding Bobbi, staring at the clumps of blood on the floor. The sudden silence made him feel sick. *What the fuck just happened?* he thought.

Paul doesn't know how long he sat in the birthing suite on his own. No-one told him what was happening or what he should be doing for Bobbi. He knew she had to feed, and that

I had already expressed milk for her, so he asked a nurse to help him find the bottle. While Bobbi was feeding, he asked the nurse, 'What's going on with my wife?'

The nurse didn't say anything. Her silence made him feel even sicker.

'There was a complication and Chloe had to be rushed to the ER,' someone eventually told Paul. I was having emergency surgery. They couldn't tell him if I was going to be okay.

In the theatre downstairs, I was thirstier than I had ever been. I desperately needed a sip of water. I begged the anaesthetist for a drink – a drop! – of water. My mouth was so parched, I thought I was going to vomit, but the anaesthetist flat-out refused. 'You can't have water; you're being put under.' He was blunt and, frankly, rude. He kept asking me the same questions: 'What's your full name and your date of birth?' He pushed me to answer. I can't remember doing so, but I must have. I closed my eyes and told myself I just had to hold on for a few more minutes, then they'd knock me out and I would stop feeling thirsty. I'd stop feeling everything. *Just close your eyes, Chloe,* I thought.

As I was closing my eyes, Paul was wiping his. He was beside himself. It wasn't until Clare came back from the ER that Paul found out what was happening. 'Chloe's lost a lot of blood,' she told him. 'When the placenta ripped off from the uterus, the lining of the uterus should have clotted and started to heal, but Chloe's didn't. She's bleeding internally, that's why we had to take her away so quickly.'

Time passed and stood still. Paul left the birthing suite with Bobbi and settled in our hospital room. He felt alone and helpless. On the outside, he was trying to keep it together for our newborn baby, but on the inside, he was a mess. *Surely the world can't be so cruel, to take such a beautiful woman away after delivering the baby she's dreamed about all her life,* he thought.

For a second, he pictured his life without me, raising Bobbi on his own. He couldn't bear the thought of me not being there to cherish the baby we had tried so hard for. Paul's fear spiral was interrupted by the sound of a phone ringing.

My phone wouldn't stop buzzing. My mum was understandably chasing updates, but I wasn't there to answer it. And Paul had his hands full. He called Ell and asked her to come back to the hospital. 'I need your help, Ell,' he said. 'Chloe's mum keeps ringing, and I don't know what to say. I don't even know what's going on.'

Ell came back and sat with Paul and Bobbi. They were uncharacteristically quiet. Just like Paul, Ell couldn't bear the thought of me dying, so she didn't even entertain it. She'd already lost one soulmate; she couldn't lose another. 'She'll be right,' Ell said to Paul.

'Are you sure?' Paul asked.

Ell paused. She wasn't. She lied. 'Yes, I'm sure. She's going to be okay,' she bluffed. 'You know how tough she is.'

My Happy Meal went cold.

At 4 pm, a nurse told Paul that I was out of surgery and in ICU. 'She's okay,' the nurse explained as she brought Paul and Bobbi to see me. 'It was a tricky situation. If we'd left it three minutes longer, she wouldn't have made it.'

The anaesthetist wasn't being rude to me, he was doing his job. He needed me to tell him my name and date of birth so he could put me under. He didn't have time to argue about my thirst. He had seconds to help save my life.

I had experienced a postpartum haemorrhage. For a vaginal birth, a blood loss of anything under 500 mL is considered normal. By the time I was taken to theatre for surgery, I had lost 1650 mL of blood. After surgery, the loss was over 2000 mL – nearly half of all the blood in my body. Like the nurse said, I was lucky to be alive. I had been minutes away from death.

In theatre, I was given two blood transfusions. The stitches I had just been given were cut open. The doctors and nurses pulled more clumps of blood out of me with their hands. Then they inserted a balloon into my uterus to help stop the bleeding and let it heal.

When I woke up in the ICU, I promptly spewed my guts up. The pressure was so great, vomit came out of my nose. It was disgusting. And painful. I wanted to cough up chunks of vomit from my throat, but I couldn't do that without busting the stitches in my vagina. I felt wet underneath, but I had a catheter in so I couldn't have weed myself. I asked a nurse if I'd shit myself. She assured me that I hadn't, but I don't know whether she was telling me the truth.

I woke up alone. 'Where is my husband?' I asked. 'Where is my baby? I need my husband, I need him, I need him,' I begged.

When I finally saw Paul, he was wearing my fluffy pink dressing gown and his bucket hat. I needed him and he was there, like a vision. He came in holding Bobbi. It was so amazing to see Paul and our baby girl. I tried to smile, but I was too out of it.

Paul later told me that I looked half dead. I had tubes and cords hooked up all over me. 'It was the gnarliest I've ever seen you, and I've seen you come out of heaps of surgeries and procedures,' he said.

Of course, he didn't say any of that in the moment. He just rubbed my head and held my hand. When the nurses told Paul to put Bobbi on my boob to feed, he thought they were joking. 'Are you kidding? This chick's half dead,' he said.

They weren't kidding. Somehow, Bobbi latched onto my boob, and I fed her in my out-of-it state. Paul was in complete awe. He called me Wonder Woman. He couldn't believe what my body had been through in the last twenty-four hours – let alone the last four and a half years – and that I was still able to breastfeed our baby.

The female body is truly, completely and utterly amazing.

I needed to speak to my mum. I didn't have my phone on me, so I asked a nurse if I could use the 'home phone'. I must have forgotten the word for 'landline.' I needed to let Mum know what had happened. No-one had told her. She'd arrived at our place on the Goldy, and had been asking Paul and Ell nonstop if I'd had the baby, if it was a boy or girl, if I was okay, what the hell was going on. Paul didn't have the capacity to answer, and Ell felt that it wasn't her place. It was an awkward position for Ell to be in; she understood how excited and worried my mum would have been, but she also knew that she couldn't be the one to give the update. Bobbi was my news to share. I had to be the one to tell my mum she was a grandmother.

'I need you to come here right now,' I said to Mum when I called her late that night. She was at my side in a flash. The nurses brought Bobbi back down from the maternity ward, so I got to introduce her to her nan. 'Mum, meet Bobbi.'

We gave Bobbi the same middle name as mine and Mum's: Maree. The name united us all. There we were, three generations of women together. Few words were spoken; none were needed. Mum hugged me and held Bobbi, the newest branch in our family tree. It was so sweet.

When Ell went to bed the night Bobbi was born, knowing I was okay and in safe hands, she said she fell asleep with a smile on her face. *Everything is right in the world,* she thought. *This is how it was meant to be.*

Meanwhile, back at the hospital, I spent my first night as a mother in the ICU, away from my baby. Every couple of hours, the nurses would wheel Bobbi down in her portable crib to feed. They helped me to hand-express milk for her to take back upstairs. I felt so lucky that my milk had come in and that Bobbi latched straight away and fed well. I was still pretty out of it, so I don't know how I would have coped if she struggled to feed.

It was almost bittersweet. I had waited so long to meet my baby, and when I finally did, I was too medicated and dozy to be present. Still, it was so much more sweet than bitter, because Bobbi was finally here. She made everything better.

I was taken back up to the maternity ward at around 11 am the next day. As I was being wheeled into the room, I saw Paul's mum at the door. She hadn't heard from either Paul or me since I went into labour two days earlier, and she was understandably worried. It had been so hectic that Paul hadn't had a chance to call her – he didn't know what to say while I was in ICU. 'I didn't want to invade your privacy, but I hadn't heard from anyone, and I needed to know if you were okay,' she said. My heart broke that she'd been sitting in such uncertainty.

It was special that Paul's mum got to meet Bobbi with him, just as my mum had done with me the night before. Both nannas were absolutely smitten. So was I. Bobbi was the most precious thing in the world. I wanted to bottle every moment with her; every yawn, every blink, every move she made.

When I returned to the maternity ward, I was taken to the delivery suite where I had given birth less than twenty-four hours earlier. 'Okay, you can hop up and have a shower and go to the toilet now that your catheter is out,' the nurse told me.

'Huh?' I was confused. I didn't know if I could use my legs; I hadn't stood up since before the epidural. Since then, I'd had anaesthesia and two blood transfusions. I'd been given countless stitches and had a catheter inserted and removed. I felt super weak and fatigued, as you would expect. It takes a while for the blood to cycle through the body and regenerate. Physically, I was frail. Mentally, I was even more fragile.

Somehow, I showered. The water washed over me. It didn't soothe me, though.

All I wanted was to be with Paul and Bobbi. I didn't want to face the outside world or speak to anyone else. I couldn't process what I'd experienced myself, and I certainly didn't have the words to explain it to others. I had birthed new life and nearly lost my own in the space of an afternoon. I didn't want to relive my near-death experience. I only wanted to stare at my baby.

I knew I had every right to crawl into the baby bubble and shut out everything else, but I felt an enormous amount of pressure to update people and answer messages and calls because so many people were invested and had sent messages of support. Everyone wanted to know about the baby and when they could meet her. I know my mum really struggled with not being there every second, but I felt like I was struggling to stay alive.

Two days after Bobbi was born, we announced her arrival on Instagram, sharing some of the beautiful photos Karina had taken in the delivery suite. I wrote:

HELLO WORLD, meet our baby girl.
Bobbi Maree Fisher.
Born 20 June 2024.
"The happiest day of the year."

If we thought our phones were blowing up before the announcement, we were in for an awakening. The response to Bobbi's birth announcement was out of this world. Friends, acquaintances and strangers alike were thrilled for us; just like they had been when we announced our pregnancy. The outpouring of support was extraordinary, but I couldn't take any of it in. I couldn't keep up with the messages. I put my phone away and tuned everything out. I had to focus – on my baby and myself.

The day after the announcement, I was sitting in my hospital bed when a nurse noticed that the colour had drained from my face once more. My colour hadn't properly returned yet, but somehow, I became even paler. It was like deja vu. When a nurse took my blood pressure, it was low. Way too low. I was taken down to the oncology ward – where cancer patients had their chemo and radiotherapy treatments – and given a blood transfusion and iron infusion.

I had a deep purple bruise on my wrist, where the doctors and nurses had tried to insert an IV before my surgery. Because I'd lost so much blood and was dehydrated, my veins had shrunk and were near-impossible to find. They would have been frantically inserting needles into my arm like a pin cushion. The bruise was a tiny glimpse of the trauma my body had gone through.

I was looking for something purple and sparkly when I saw the cowboy boots. Lilac and glitter. They had Minnie's name written all over them. Paul and I wanted to give Minnie a gift from Bobbi when she was born. We had researched the best ways to prepare children for a new baby, and one tip suggested giving the child a small gift from the baby to make them feel special. I was conscious of the bond both Paul and I shared with Minnie. She felt like our firstborn, and we wanted her to know how much we loved her, and that we always would. The boots were a small symbol of that.

As usual, I heard Minnie before I saw her. She came bouncing into the hospital room, wearing her favourite yellow crocheted set with her hair in space buns on either side of her head. She was carrying a bunch of flowers above her head like the Olympic torch. She looked so cute and proud. When Minnie chucked the flowers down, she immediately spotted her wrapped present. She didn't really clock the tiny baby in my arms; we had to point Bobbi out to her. We'd explained to Minnie that I was pregnant, and she knew there had been a baby in my tummy – she loved my big belly – but I don't think she quite understood that Bobbi was the baby who had been in my tummy.

When Minnie opened her present, we explained that Bobbi had bought her the pair of sparkly boots. 'Thank you Bobbi,' she said in her sweet little voice.

Ell sat behind Minnie as she held Bobbi for the first time. 'This is your baby sister,' Ell explained, through tears. She cried the entire visit. It was super emotional for her. She'd been with us from the beginning of our fertility journey – our grief was the thing that had really brought us together – and now her baby was holding our baby. We always imagined we would raise our kids together on the Goldy, and now it was finally happening.

Minnie kept adorably patting Bobbi on the head and saying, 'Hello.' It was the most darling moment – and one we had been so excited for – but when I try to remember it now, it's a bit of a blur. Things were hazy for me then, and they're even hazier now that time has passed.

Thank God we took so many videos and photos to look back on. Minnie put her boots on straight away and didn't take them off for a good six months. They were her 'Bobbi Boots' and she loved them dearly.

When the birth doesn't go to plan

(AND YOU'RE LEFT HOLDING MORE THAN JUST A BABY)

Birth is wild.

Even when you get a happy ending, the ride to get there can leave you completely shattered. If you've just come out the other side of a birth that left you dazed, rattled, stitched up or silent – this part is for you.

You can feel both the magic and the mess.

You can be head over heels in love with your baby and still grieving the birth you hoped for. That doesn't make you ungrateful – it makes you human.

If you're anything like me, the shock might not hit straight away.

You might feel okay in the moment, only for it to catch up with you days, weeks, or months later. That's normal. Trauma doesn't always scream; sometimes it whispers. Remember, healing isn't linear, and it doesn't follow a schedule. It takes time.

I wish someone told me this earlier: 'You don't owe anyone an update.'

The texts, the DMs, the 'when can we visit?' messages – ignore them. Your only job right now is to rest, heal, and stare at your baby (or just sleep). Your family, friends and the rest of the world can wait until YOU are ready.

Let's talk about feeding (because not enough people do).

Feeding looks different for everyone. Some babies latch straight away. Some need help.

Some parents pump. Some mix feed. Some switch to formula and find it a better fit.

Others, like me, find themselves breastfeeding for the first time while still hooked up to tubes, half-conscious in ICU, wondering how the hell their body is even functioning – let alone feeding a baby.

None of it is easy.

None of it is wrong.

We're made to believe that there's a 'right way' to feed your baby. That breastfeeding is the ultimate gold standard. That formula is a back-up plan. That pumping is exhausting but noble. That you should be able to just 'push through' if it hurts, if your nipples bleed, if you have a blocked milk duct. After all, it's what's best for the baby.

Here's the truth.

The right way to feed your baby is the way that works for you.

The one that lets *you* heal. The one that allows your baby to grow. The one that honours both of your needs.

And if your feeding journey hasn't looked like the one you imagined?

If you've cried into your breast pads or stared at a bottle feeling guilty or frustrated or confused – you are not alone.

Feeding isn't just physical. It's emotional. It's hormonal. It's personal. It can bring up *all* the things – fear, failure, frustration, grief, even trauma.

So, wherever you are on your journey, whether it's your first feed or your fiftieth time questioning yourself, please remember this . . .

You are feeding your baby with love.

And that, Mumma, is enough.

The body remembers its old self and will slowly return.

Don't be surprised if you're sore for longer than expected. Blood loss, surgery, transfusions – your body's been through the wringer. Be gentle. You just did the impossible.

It was months after I had Bobbi that I felt a bulge inside my vagina. I'd briefly read about vaginal prolapses, but I hadn't heard anyone openly speak about them. So I'm speaking about them here. A prolapse is a condition where the bladder, uterus and/or bowel protrudes into the vagina when the tissues and muscles in your pelvis weaken and overstretch. I went to see a pelvic floor physio and I was given a pessary – a removable, flexible device inserted into the vagina – to support my pelvic organs. Thankfully, my prolapse was only minor and gradually fixed itself, and I no longer have to wear the pessary.

There's no such thing as a textbook recovery from childbirth. Bodies don't just 'bounce back'. It takes time, support and often professional help.

Your mind needs time to heal, too.

After something as momentous as giving birth (or nearly losing your life while doing it), your body doesn't just need to heal, your mind does too.

In the weeks after Bobbi's birth, I found myself replaying moments on loop. The silence in the birthing suite. The emergency button. Paul's kiss on my forehead. That terrifying question to my midwife, Lisa: 'Am I dying?'

I felt like I should have been in the baby bubble, but my brain kept dragging me back to the trauma.

A few weeks later, when I felt ready, Paul and I sat down with my midwives Lisa and Clare for a birth debrief. They walked me through every step of what happened, down to the minute, both medically and emotionally. They explained the moments I couldn't remember clearly. It was confronting, but also incredibly healing.

I finally understood the reason behind the chaos, which helped me feel like I could start piecing things together.

If you've been through a traumatic birth or felt disconnected from your experience, you deserve that space too. Ask your midwife or hospital about doing a birth debrief. Talk to someone. Write it out. Cry if you need to.

Take the photo anyway.

Even if you feel half dead, bloated or blank – take it. One day, you'll look back and see a warrior woman. Even if you don't recognise her just yet.

Even in the haze, you did it.

You birthed a baby.

You birthed a new version of yourself.

And I promise – she's magic too.

– Source unknown

Seventeen

THE FUTURE IS NOW

I DIDN'T WANT TO LEAVE THE HOSPITAL. I WAS HAPPY TO BE there, in the cocoon of our room, in the safe hands of trained professionals. Because of my postpartum haemorrhage, I spent a week in the hospital following Bobbi's birth. During that time, the midwives and nurses took such amazing care of me – those people are genuinely angels on earth. I couldn't have survived the first week of motherhood without them, and I mean that quite literally. After my first visit to the oncology ward, I had to go back for another blood transfusion and iron infusion days later.

Walking out of the maternity ward to take Bobbi home was hard, and not just because I could barely walk. I think the nurses and midwives were sad to see us go, too. Bobbi was such a good baby, and they adored her. I swear she got cuter every day. Her cheeks got chubbier, and her eyelashes grew longer. People said she looked like a little doll. She sounded like one, too – she barely ever cried. I wondered where her chilled energy came from.

When we got home, I burst into heavy sobs. I was in agony walking up the stairs to our second floor. The stitches between my vagina and bum pulsed with pain. I had very little relief because I was adamant about getting off painkillers as soon as possible. I didn't want to fuck around with opioids. I knew how troubling they could be. By that point, I'd had enough procedures – laparoscopies, hysteroscopies, corrective surgery on my broken wrist and the Asherman's operation – to know how painkillers affected me. One of my biggest concerns after the birth was that the tablets would make me constipated. I weaned off the meds, took laxatives and drank prune juice. None of it helped.

Our first night at home was a total shitshow. In every sense. Bobbi was feeding every couple of hours, so Paul and I were tag-teaming. I was feeding, while Paul did the nappy changing. In the darkest hour of the night, I was sitting on the toilet with the breast pump attached to my boobs, crying because the wee was stinging my stitches. Paul was changing Bobbi on the change mat on the dresser of our bedroom. He lifted her legs to put a new nappy underneath her, and Bobbi promptly exploded with poo. I swear, it shot two metres across the room. It was bright orange, and it was all over our brand-new white carpet. Paul – the clean freak – tried to scrub it out, but that just made it worse. He was beyond stressed and couldn't sleep the rest of the night, not because of Bobbi waking every two hours but because of his precious carpet . . .

When Ell called in the morning to see how our first night had gone, I asked if she could pretty-please organise for a carpet cleaner to come to our place. Ell nailed the brief – instead of bringing us a meal, she brought us carpet cleaners.

We felt entirely out of our depth. I started to wonder why we'd been allowed to leave the hospital with this baby when we had absolutely no idea what we were doing!

While Bobbi was pooing freely, I was not. I was so scared to shit. I remember being on the toilet and begging for someone to help me. I couldn't strain because of my stitches, and even though I needed to poo, I wasn't able to. It got so bad, Clare – who was kindly doing my postpartum care at home out of the goodness of her heart, bless her – had to come over that day to give me an enema. Clare remembers thinking I looked broken. That's exactly how I felt.

When I finally pooed, I predictably split my stitches open. It was horrendous. My voice still trembles when I talk about it now. I went back to hospital, and I was taken into the same delivery suite to get stitched back up. The trauma was real. I was given a shot of local anaesthetic, and my obstetrician gave me new stitches, for at least the third time.

I was sure I was never going to recover. I couldn't see how I would ever walk, sit or poo normally again. I definitely couldn't imagine having sex ever again. The pain was so relentless and intense, I felt like I was outside of my body. The only time I wasn't in agony was when I was sleeping. And I wasn't doing much of that.

It was hard to enjoy my first weeks of motherhood – the only thing I've ever wanted – because of the intense pain I was in. And yet, I still did. The only thing that made any of it bearable was Bobbi. She was such a good girl. An angel. She slept really well, fed smoothly and rarely cried. I don't know how I would have coped if she was unsettled or had colic or reflux.

In that sense – and so many others – Bobbi was a blessing. I held her in my arms as I stood at the front door and waved goodbye to Paul at the end of June. He had to leave us to start his residency in Ibiza. Bobbi was sixteen days old. We'd only had nine days at home as a family of three. Conscious of our limited time together, I wanted Paul and Bobbi to bond as much as they possibly could. Once again, I felt like crawling into a cocoon and blocking out the rest of the world.

I know some people in our lives found that hard. I felt like I spent a lot of my limited time and energy worrying about other people's feelings. I was so depleted that I didn't have the energy to give to anyone except Bobbi. The focus should have been on Bobbi and my recovery, but it was shifted to upset feelings. I didn't need that block of guilt added to my Jenga tower of emotions. I was sure it would topple me.

I bawled my eyes out when Paul left. So did he. It was heavy. Paul had to force himself to get in the car and drive away. I watched as the car left our driveway and my whole world drove off into the distance. *What the fuck am I going to do?* I wondered. *I have a little baby to keep alive, but I can barely keep myself alive right now.*

It's true what they say: it takes a village to raise a child. As soon as Paul left, my mum came to help out. Ellidy, Laura and our good friend Tiana were always close by, and Paul's best mate, Kane, would drop off home-cooked meals for me every night. He had made me a hearty stew when I was still in hospital after my haemorrhage, and it was one of the best things I've ever eaten.

As well as my Goldy family, Olivia and Lachie also came up from Sydney to stay for a week. Olivia especially was a godsend, because she's a nurse.

My sister definitely saw a different side to me when I was postpartum. Olivia has described me as being polished and organised. I was neither of those things. I felt like I was falling apart. I remember asking Liv to check me out when my stitches started to come out; it felt like I had a gaping hole between my vagina and bum. The pain I was in outweighed any shame I might have felt showing my sister the mess that was in between my legs – and asking her to give me an enema. Liv was such a trooper. I could not have managed without her, or Lachie. We quickly slipped into a little routine.

Every morning, Lachie would do the early shift because he woke up at the same time as Bobbi. Our guest room was opposite Bobbi's nursery, so Lachie would grab Bobbi when she woke up and make her a bottle. Then he'd take her for a little walk so I could keep sleeping. They were so helpful. 'She's just the best thing that's ever happened,' Liv said about Bobbi. 'She's such a joy.'

That was exactly how I felt, too.

On the spare pages at the back of my pregnancy journal, Ellidy and Laura wrote notes to Bobbi. *Hello little pumpkin, I can't wait to cuddle you and watch you grow into the most loved little being. Minnie and I promise to be your best friends forever! We are going to have so so so many fun adventures together little bubba. We love you so much already,* Ell wrote from her and Minnie.

Oh Bobbi girl!!! You are HERE. Ahhh. You are so so loved and melting our hearts daily. I know you know your journey getting here was a wild one . . . Looking in your beautiful eyes I can tell you are a wise, sweet, special little soul. I can't wait to watch you grow. Your mum and dad are the best. Love you forever, Aunty Lala, added Laura.

We asked Ellidy and Laura to be Bobbi's godmothers, and Kane to be her godfather.

The outpouring of love for Bobbi was so beautiful. Minnie was especially enamoured with her little sister. Ellidy would put Minnie in the car and say, 'We're going to Coco's!'

'Bobbi! We get to see Bobbi!' Minnie would reply.

Ell caught her in the back seat talking to herself one day. 'Be gentle, be gentle,' Minnie was saying to herself, repeating what we would tell her when she was cuddling the baby. When they got to our place, Minnie would run inside – usually wearing her sparkly purple cowboy boots – saying, 'Can I hold it? Can I hold it?'

Seeing Minnie and Bobbi together was so special. I remember all those months – years – I'd imagined me and Ell raising our kids as besties, and it was finally happening. Our future was now.

I tried to hold onto that knowledge, but some days I couldn't find comfort in it. As hard as it was falling pregnant and giving birth, by far the hardest thing for me was postpartum. Being a mum was *so* much harder than I'd ever imagined.

I remember messaging Paul in the middle of the night saying, *I'm really struggling. Bobbi won't sleep, I can't get her to burp, I know she's not hungry, I don't know what to do. I'm so tired.*

I know part of my struggle was my arduous recovery following the birth, episiotomy and postpartum haemorrhage. The other part was the relentlessness of motherhood. It's constant. There are no breaks. And definitely no sick days.

There were so many times when I just wanted to press pause and take a deep breath, but there's no remote control for life. I couldn't pause the milk squirting out of my boobs. I couldn't pause the shit leaking out of Bobbi's nappy. I couldn't pause the world to get the sleep I needed.

I was finally a mum – the only role I'd ever wanted – but I didn't feel human anymore.

I was afraid to leave the house. I couldn't see myself ever being able to go outside again. How could I? My body had been torn apart, and my baby was tiny. We couldn't just walk out the front door.

I thought there was something deeply wrong with me; that I was broken.

It was Ell who first mentioned the words 'baby blues'. I had heard of postpartum depression before because a friend had gone through it, but I didn't think that was what I was experiencing. I googled 'baby blues' and read the definition: 'A common, temporary experience of mood swings, tearfulness and anxiety that many new mothers experience in the first few days or weeks after childbirth, typically due to hormonal changes.'

I ticked all the boxes. The main difference between postpartum depression and baby blues is that the latter is temporary, while the former is more serious and persistent. Knowing that the baby blues was a common – and temporary – occurrence put me at ease a little.

It was a reminder that when it comes to mental health, some things are out of our control. There was nothing wrong with me; there was a hormonal imbalance in my brain that made me incredibly sad and scared to leave the house. I was reminded again of the panic attacks I'd had as a teenager, and the knowledge that mental health issues don't discriminate. I had everything I ever wanted in Bobbi, and I still experienced the baby blues. It had nothing to do with my circumstances, and everything to do with my hormones and the chemicals in my brain.

I rode the hormonal wave and got smashed by a few dumpers. But with the help of my loved ones, I managed to keep my head above water.

Bobbi and I had our first proper outing with Mum and Olivia. We went to a nearby cafe and Bobbi screamed the whole drive there – she wasn't a fan of the car. In the end, I spent more time getting Bobbi ready, preparing her bottles and packing the baby bag than we did at the cafe. It was such an ordeal just to get out the front door.

I was still in a dark place when I recorded my birth story for *Darling, Shine!* The bruises were still on my wrist from where they'd tried to cannulate my dehydrated veins. I was open and honest about my labour journey, but I wasn't ready to share what had happened to me after giving birth to Bobbi. I knew our *Darling, Shine!* listeners were so excited to hear about Bobbi and her arrival – they had been on the fertility journey with me the whole way – and I didn't want to end the story on such a scary note. I also didn't want anyone to think I was complaining about birth – I was so grateful for the experience. Mostly, though, I just didn't know what to say. I was still processing it all myself.

The one thing I definitely wanted to say was thank you to Paul. 'Your support throughout my labour was a testament to the incredible partner and father you are. In those intense moments, your strength became my anchor, your calm my solace. Watching you stand by my side, feeling your hand in mine, I was reminded of the depth of our bond and the unbreakable love that we share. You were my rock when I needed it most and I can't thank you enough for being there every step of the way,' I said. 'My love for you is like no other. Together we have faced challenges and celebrated triumphs, but nothing compares to the experience of bringing our daughter into this world with you by my side. You are my partner, my best friend, and now the most amazing father to our child. I love you more than words can express, and I am so grateful for the life we have built together.'

At the four-week appointment with my obstetrician, he said we needed to talk about contraception. 'You know the best contraception? Labour,' I quipped. I couldn't even begin to imagine having sex again. I didn't want anything near my vagina. And I couldn't see that changing.

Ell said she noticed the colour coming back into my face at around the four-week mark. It wasn't until I was seven weeks postpartum, though, that I started to feel like myself again. I was in a pale haze until then. I had definitely lost who I was.

My return to self came just in time. At the start of August, Bobbi and I were set to fly to LA to meet Paul and travel back to Ibiza with him. Bobbi's first ever flight was from the Gold Coast to Sydney. Both my mum and dad came up for the occasion and to help me on the ninety-minute flight. On that flight, I thought, *How do people do this on their own? How the hell did Ellidy fly with Minnie to the other side of the world? How did she do a wee without someone with her to hold Minnie?*

Once again, I was in awe of Ell, her independence and grace.

I spent a couple of nights in Sydney with my parents to break up the trip. My mum couldn't believe how smiley Bobbi was. 'You never smiled as a baby,' she told me.

Bobbi kept smiling on our way to LAX. My friend Bianca joined us on the flight to give me a hand. Both she and Bobbi were legends. I had been understandably nervous about travelling with a baby, but the flight was relatively pain-free. And it was all worth it when we saw Paul at the other end.

Paul scooped us up in his arms and I never wanted him to let go. Seeing him as a dad was pure magic. Paul was obsessed with Bobbi. I know I'm biased, but he is the most doting dad in the entire universe. Paul always said he wanted to be a present, hands-on and fun father, and that's exactly what he is. He loves one-on-one time with Bobbi, and that's one of the reasons I was committed to pumping, so Paul could bottle-feed her.

Bobbi had grown so much in the five weeks Paul was away, he couldn't believe it. She was so much more awake to the world and her little personality was already bursting through. He missed her so much – almost as much as we'd missed him. At his show at Day Trip Festival in LA someone had made a sign with a photo of the three of us and the words: 'The world held on for Bobbi.' It was a nod to Paul's remix of 'World, Hold On'. There were also signs with my face, Ellidy's and Minnie's. Our little modern family.

My reunion with Paul in LA was lovely, but a little chaotic. It wasn't until we got to Ibiza a few days later that we could really settle into being a family of three.

I spent my thirty-third birthday in Spain, with my husband, baby and a handful of close friends. I ate oysters for lunch and breastfed Bobbi out of the Mediterranean sun. My daughter looked up at me with her big, wide eyes and my heart burst. It was the best birthday I've ever had.

How to support new parents

Advice for loved ones

RESPECT BOUNDARIES

New parenthood is a special time, but it can also be difficult, confronting and challenging. It's important to listen to the wishes of Mum and Dad, and act accordingly. If they say they don't want visitors at the hospital or in the first couple of weeks at home, respect that. If they ask for people to call before rocking up, respect that. If they say they need time alone as a family unit, respect that.

FOLLOW THEIR LEAD

It's basic social media etiquette to wait for the parents to announce the arrival of their new baby. After all, it's their news to share. We know how tempting it is to share photos of an adorable newborn, but everyone should check in with the parents before doing so.

GIVE TIME, SPACE AND GRACE

It's difficult to see clearly in the postpartum fog. Don't blame new parents if they take weeks to reply to a message or forget to call you back. The fourth trimester can be rough, and the last thing people with a new baby need is pressure and guilt. Try to be understanding, and give grace instead of guilt.

BE PRACTICAL

Flowers are a lovely gesture, but you know what's better than a gesture for someone with a newborn? A home-cooked meal, a set of clean sheets on their bed, an offer to wash up, or a folded basket of washing. The most supportive thing you can do for new parents is to be practical and provide support.

SAFETY FIRST

It should go without saying, but visitors should refrain from kissing the newborn – no matter how squishy their cheeks are. When babies are born, their immune system is not fully developed, so they have a higher risk of catching an infection. Be conscious of that, make sure your whooping cough vaccinations are up to date, and avoid visiting if you're feeling unwell.

TAKE NOTE

As I've said, the baby blues are common, and they don't discriminate, but they are temporary. If a new mum continues to feel sad, anxious or overwhelmed for a prolonged period, it could be a sign of postpartum depression (PPD). There is help and support for PPD, if it is recognised. Therapy and medication can make a real difference. It's important for the loved ones of new mums to take note of PPD signs and know that help is available.

Eighteen

LETTING GO

'Once you hold your baby in your arms, all the heartache will feel like a distant memory,' people used to tell me when I was in the thick of pregnancy loss. I couldn't see how it was true. The heartache felt inescapable. It was suffocating.

For almost five years, my life felt heavy. The weight of miscarriage and infertility wore me down. But those people were right. As soon as Bobbi arrived, that heaviness lifted. I felt light.

I still have trauma from my pregnancy losses, but having Bobbi has eased the pain. She has righted so many wrongs. I can look back on our journey and clearly see that she was meant to be. Bobbi was waiting in the wings to make her arrival at just the right time. She was a miracle.

For the first time, I was able to stick a polaroid in the back of my pregnancy journal in 2024. It was a photo of me and Paul, sitting on our couch at home, holding a newborn Bobbi.

I started to reflect on my lost pregnancies and wondered if they had happened for a reason. I thought that reason might have been so we could pour our love and energy into Ell and Minnie. If Paul and I had a child of our own when Minnie was a baby, we wouldn't have had the same bond with her. Of course, we still would have been in her life, but she wouldn't have had our undivided attention.

'It was like Bobbi was waiting for the right moment to come into our life,' I told Ell on a podcast episode. 'I do believe that maybe our other babies didn't come because it was our opportunity to be there for you and be there for Minnie Moo – and give her those beautiful, solid years of one-on-one time with her.'

The universe had a plan for us. I knew that, even if I didn't always trust it. I should have trusted it.

I used to tell myself that my story was already written – 'whatever will be, will be' – but I had no idea just how incredible the story was going to get.

Our 2024 summer in Ibiza was like no other. We'd spent the last two visits there with Ellidy and Minnie. This time around, me and Ell did a full role reversal. I was the one with a little baby, breastfeeding and trying to catch some sleep, while she was the one solo, staying out late and sleeping in.

I was the one on antibiotics for mastitis; she was the one doing tequila shots. Ell was only on the ground in Ibiza for six days, so Minnie stayed at home with my mum. It sucked for us, because we didn't get to hang out with her, but it was great for Ell, who needed – and deserved – a break.

There was another reason for Ell's whirlwind trip . . . Laura was (secretly) getting married to her childhood sweetheart, Jake. Laura, Jake and I had all gone to primary school together, so we'd been in each other's lives for as long as we could make memories. We'd grown up beside each other, and now I was going to stand beside Laura and Jake on their wedding day. The Baby Spice to my Sporty Spice was going to be a bride!

I was Laura's maid of honour, so I organised her hens' party at O Beach Day Club. Paul was excited to be on solo Bobbi duty. We took a party bus to the bar, wearing our matching cowgirl hats, and I had a Vodka Cruiser on the drive. It had been so long since I'd had an alcoholic beverage that I genuinely felt drunk from one drink. I tried to embrace the tipsiness, but I was out of practice.

At O Beach, we got a table right in the thick of the action, surrounded by music and champagne. It felt a bit like Mums Gone Wild; our friend Tash also left her kids at home to come to the destination wedding. I was enjoying having a few bevvies – and pumping and dumping my breastmilk in the bathroom. Ell being Ell drank a cup of my milk and said it tasted like Yakult. She offered some to the other girls in the bathroom, who politely declined. 'Milk doesn't really go with vodka and soda.'

Fair point.

We finished the night watching Paul's show at Hï from 3 am. I tapped out at 5 am, but everyone else kicked on. Ellidy told me later she felt liberated. It would have been one of the first times in the four years since Chumpy died, and the two and a half years since Minnie was born, that she could really let go. When you've suffered a loss, there's so much guilt. I think that guilt is amplified when you're a mum. It taints happy moments and ruins fun. It whispers in your ear: *How can you possibly be having a good time when your soulmate is gone? Or when your baby is at home? Or when you have three loads of washing to do?*

That night at Hï, Ell danced the guilt away, and it was bloody beautiful to see.

The beauty continued. Laura and Jake got married on a yacht off Es Vedrà island, where we'd spent our favourite days of the summer the past couple of years. There were only fourteen of us on the boat. It was intimate and romantic, and so fitting for Laura and Jake, who had been together for ten years.

Laura wore the most stunning sheer white Jacquemus dress with a one-piece swimsuit underneath. Watching her walk down the 'aisle' is a moment I'll remember for eternity. She almost glided toward Jake. Their vows were deep and emotional. We were all crying happy tears.

Adorably, Laura and Jake asked Bobbi to be the flower girl *and* the ring bearer. Our friend LJ was the celebrant, and she introduced Bobbi: 'I'd like to welcome Bobbi Fisher down the aisle. She has zero motor skills yet, but she's the ring bearer.' I carried Bobbi in my arms with the ring boxes resting on her belly. When we got to Laura and Jake, one of the boxes tumbled off Bobbi – and headed straight toward the ocean! LJ dived for it and hit the deck with a thud. Incredibly, she grabbed it! Everyone cheered, and pure chaos erupted. The ceremony was stopped for a good ten minutes because we were all laughing so much. It could have been a disaster, but it became one of the best parts of the day. Little Bobbi was at the centre of it.

I had to pinch myself that my baby was at my best friend's wedding. For two years in a row, I had visited Es Vedrà – home to the patron goddess of fertility – as my arms ached for a baby. And there I was, holding the baby I'd wished for in my arms.

The sun set over the Mediterranean Sea, bathing us all in a golden glow. We swam and danced and ate merrily. It was one of the best days of my life.

When we got home from the wedding, all I wanted was to curl up in bed. Instead, I showered Bobbi, pumped and dumped my breastmilk, sanitised her bottles, made formula bottles for the night, washed my breast pump, and got the baby to sleep. They reckon a mother's job is never done, and they're right (whoever they are).

The week of Laura and Jake's wedding was epic. Our closest friends were in Ibiza and on a high to be celebrating the beautiful couple. I was determined to be present and enjoy every moment, but I wasn't always able to do that. The villa where all our mates were staying was a forty-five minute drive from our home. Bobbi would cry the whole way there and back. I couldn't handle the sound of her crying; it was torturous. She was always completely fine as soon as we got her out of the car, but her tears made even quick trips painful for me.

Ell had a theory about babies crying. 'They just need to let their emotions out,' she told me. 'Sometimes it's good to have a cry.'

I certainly felt like crying. And I did. I couldn't help but burst into tears a number of times over the week. I felt overwhelmed, anxious and on edge. I couldn't relax. I wanted to do *all the things* with my friends, but I also wanted to spend every second with my baby. I had organised for some help from a nanny – which I know is a privileged thing to be able to do – but trying to juggle that was exhausting in itself. My emotions went into overdrive, and my hormones hit the accelerator. I was bound to crash.

For a moment, I was worried I had the baby blues again. Paul kept asking me what was wrong, and I was tempted to give him a list. The main thing was obviously that I was running on empty and putting too much pressure on myself. I didn't want to ruin the mood with all my crying, but trying to plaster on a smile was making me want to cry more. I needed to let go. I needed to channel my inner Ell on the dance floor at Hï at 3 am.

I don't want any of this to come across as complaining. I'm not having a whinge; I'm sharing my reality. I know our time in Ibiza looked amazing on Instagram – and it genuinely was amazing – but nothing is picture-perfect. Underneath the glossy images, I was a new mum, going through so many emotional, hormonal and physical changes.

In the past, when I've shared some of my struggles on the podcast, we got comments like: 'You ungrateful little brat. Your life is perfect. You have no right to complain. How privileged of you.' There are entire Reddit threads dedicated to hating on me and Ell. Someone literally posted a question on the 'ausinfluencersnark' Reddit asking, 'Thoughts on Ellidy and Chloe partying it up in Ibiza like they are twenty-one?'

Even though I know it's a pile of internalised misogynistic bullshit, it still burns. For someone like me, who has always strived to be good – a good student, a good worker, a good human – the criticism got under my skin.

It took me a long time to realise I can't please everyone. I'm damned if I do, damned if I don't. If I speak about the good times, I'm showing off. If I speak about the hard days, I'm a spoiled bitch. I can't win. All I can do is stop reading the comments and keep it real – because no-one's life is perfect, and it's fucked up to pretend that it is.

After 'partying it up in Ibiza like we're twenty-one', Ellidy, Minnie, Paul, Bobbi and I went on our first holiday as a family of five to New York in October 2024. Paul and I were as excited as ever to see Minnie Moo. In the same way I loved watching Paul with Minnie, I loved watching Bobbi with her too. I swear she lights up when Minnie walks into the room.

The gang was back together. We were walking around the streets of the Big Apple, wearing 'I ♥ NY' tees, going to the Museum of Ice Cream and eating bagels. And naturally, we were posting about our adventures on the *Darling, Shine!* Instagram account. That's when we started getting messages. *Omg, I'm in NYC, I'd love to meet you guys,* one of our followers wrote. Then another. And another.

'We should do a meet-and-greet,' I said to Ell. It wasn't something I had ever suggested before – namely because I was too afraid no-one would show up.

We threw caution – and our imposter syndrome – to the wind and put out a time to meet up in Central Park. We thought maybe five people would turn up, and that would be lovely. I still had a sinking feeling that no-one would come. Like, who the hell did we think we were? Who would want to meet us? Especially here, on the other side of the world from our homeland?

Ell, Minnie and I got to Central Park five minutes late, and when we rounded the corner to the meet-up spot, there was a crowd. There must have been over fifty people waiting for us. Ellidy ran straight toward the group, and I got suddenly shy. It was staggering, in the loveliest way possible.

There were cuddles and tears and stories. The women – and the few guys who came – were genuine and friendly, and so like-minded. It felt like we were all mates, even though we were meeting for the first time. It was so wholesome. One of the girls told us she had driven eight hours to come. Another came all the way from Canada! I couldn't believe it.

We weren't used to people wanting to get selfies with us. Ell and I record the podcast in a room behind closed doors; we don't perform in front of crowds like Paul. He's the one who gets recognised and has people fangirl over him. We're usually the ones taking the photos for him. Paul had been named International DJ of the Year earlier in the month, so he was getting stopped on the street more and more.

When Paul came to the meet-and-greet with Bobbi at the end, he was blown away by how many people were there. Walking back to our hotel, he told me how proud he was of us. 'Wow, that was incredible. I can't believe how many people showed up. Look at the community you've built, it's so special,' he said to me and Ell.

Darling, Shine! had done what we set out to do: made people feel less alone in their struggles. So many of the women at the meet-up said they had been inspired by Ell and me, which was a bit strange to hear. We hadn't planned on being inspirational, we were just being ourselves and telling our stories. That's not always easy to do, so I guess in that sense, it is inspiring. The podcast resonated with people in a way we had only dreamed of.

The *Darling, Shine!* meet-up was the unexpected highlight of the trip. Truth be told, I thought it was going to be *The Lion King*. We'd bought tickets to the Broadway musical as a surprise for Minnie (and organised for our beautiful Ibiza nanny to come to New York to look after Bobbi). I had a vision of a wholesome family night out with me, Paul, Ell and Minnie. I thought going to the theatre in NYC would be a core childhood memory for Minnie. My vision was a little off.

Ell had had a big one the night before, and she literally fell asleep in the theatre as soon as we sat down. I'm not exaggerating; she was snoring. Meanwhile, Minnie couldn't sit still. She was playing with her Lion King toys from the gift shop and throwing the program around. I was so embarrassed, and felt so bad for the people sitting behind us. We left before intermission. That night is something Ell and I laugh about now. I doubt Minnie remembers any of the show.

She might remember another show, though . . . Paul played the We Belong Here festival in Central Park and we brought Minnie along to watch his set. Wearing a set of pink headphones and eating a stick of fairy floss, Minnie watched Paul in awe. She bopped around on people's shoulders and had an absolute ball.

Those are the moments I live for. Doing our thing with our people. After our time in New York, Ell and Minnie spent a few days with us in our LA home. We went to our favourite sushi joint, and cooked dinner at home. We bickered and teased each other – well, Ell and Paul teased me – and got on each other's nerves, as all families do. 'This has been the best part of the whole trip,' Paul said of the quality family time we had in LA.

I cried when Ell and Minnie flew back to Australia, even though I knew I would be back on the Goldy with them soon enough. Paul, Bobbi and I had a few more weeks – and a handful more shows – overseas before heading home for the Aussie summer. I was so looking forward to spending days at the beach with Bobbi.

On a particular beach day in December, Paul filmed a cheeky video to reveal his hair transplant. 'Ah, nothing like sand in my toes. . . And wind in my hair, baby!' he said to the camera, as he walked into the ocean. His hair looked great, and it got lots of attention. The tabloids ran with the headline: 'DJ Fisher doesn't look like this anymore.'

Paul wasn't shy about getting a hair transplant. He didn't mind being bald, so he wasn't sensitive about it. But the issue for him was that he wasn't completely bald. His hair still grew at the back and sides of his head, so he had to shave it off every single day with a Bic razor. It was irritating. It grew so quickly, he often had stubble by the end of the day. He was over it. He asked a laser clinic if they'd permanently laser all of his hair off, but they refused, so he went down the hair transplant route instead.

The process was hectic. Over two days and twelve hours, Paul sat in a chair while the hair transplant surgeon took follicles from the back of his head and implanted them on the top of his head. There were 8500 hair grafts all up. The surgeon said it was one of the biggest transplants he'd ever done in Australia.

The result was pretty gnarly. Paul's head swelled up like he was having a severe allergic reaction, and it was covered in what looked like ingrown hairs. It looked sore, and it was. Worst of all, Paul couldn't sleep on his head for the three nights, so he went to bed with a neck pillow, as though he was boarding a long-haul flight. Eventually, the transplanted hairs grew and fell out, and new hairs began to grow in their place. And just like that, Paul had a full head of hair.

December was for hair reveals and down time. I needed it. I felt like I was crawling to the finish line of 2024. I was feeling the strain of the year that was.

At the end of 2024, I made the difficult decision to step away from co-hosting *Darling, Shine!* full-time. Ell was ready and happy to step up and host on her own; she cleverly named her solo show *Ell, Loco.* I was still going to be a part of

Darling, Shine! and make appearances on the podcast – and, most excitingly, work on putting together a live tour – but I wasn't going to host every episode alongside Ell.

I had a bit on my plate: a baby, a jam-packed travel schedule, multiple businesses, a podcast tour to plan and a growing property development company. Paul and I officially launched YLB Properties (named after the classic Fisher track 'You Little Beauty') in early 2025. We had projects we were putting together in Bali, Ibiza and an apartment complex on the Goldy. We planned to turn the site of our first-ever home – our Palm Beach paradise – and the block next door into an eight-storey apartment building named Pescado (which means 'fish' in Spanish). We would live in the penthouse and sell the other apartments. It was an ambitious undertaking, but moving into the property development space was very exciting for me. I loved the idea of turning a vision into a reality.

My overflowing plate was just one of the reasons I decided to take time out from *Darling, Shine!* The biggest reason was a feeling of wanting to protect our community. I knew so many of the podcast listeners were people who were dealing with infertility, miscarriage and loss. They followed my story for solidarity. I could still offer that solidarity and so much empathy, but having Bobbi made me one of the lucky ones. I knew how it felt to be an unlucky one.

It's not fair. What's wrong with me? Why can't I have a baby when everyone else seems to be having one?

For years, those thoughts and questions swirled in my mind like a whirlpool, dragging me down. I didn't want to be the reason someone else asked those questions of themself.

My life now revolves around Bobbi. Being her mum is the best gig in the world, and it's a pretty all-consuming role. To share my life openly and honestly would be to talk about Bobbi every week. I want to be real and candid about this new phase of my life, but I don't want to hurt anyone in the process. As I've said, I know how hard conversations about babies can be for people trying to conceive.

On the flip side, I know some people love hearing about Bobbi. She is growing into such a bright and beautiful little girl. Sometimes I look at her and I still can't believe that she's real and she's mine. At the minute, she's a real mummy's girl, and it melts my heart when she reaches for me or smiles at me. I ran into my midwife Clare recently, and she marvelled at Bobbi. 'I thought you were photoshopping her, Chlo, but she's even cuter in real life.'

I want to share that cuteness with the world, for all the people out there who need a dose of chubby baby cheeks and adorable baby smiles. I'm working through my hesitation of talking about motherhood, and I know I'll be back on *Darling, Shine!* when the time is right. The podcast means so much to Ell and me. It's brought us closer than ever – and torn us apart a couple of times – and we're grateful for it all.

Nineteen

TIME

In many ways, Bali is where this story began. It's where I met Paul and where I started to fall for him, back when the universe kept pushing us together in 2012. Since then, Bali has been a constant in our lives. We've shared our happiest moments there: our wedding, our first holiday with Bobbi when she was six months old, and our annual family vacay with Ell and Minnie.

Bali is also where I've had my darkest days: when my grandmother passed away after our wedding, when I found out my poppa had died a couple of years later, and where I mourned the loss of my fourth miscarriage.

The thing about Bali is, it's a place of healing. Even on the worst days, Bali is a balm. It soothes. I've crumbled in Bali many times, but I've always found the strength there to piece myself back together.

My mum always said she would never go back to Bali after my grandma died there in 2020. She didn't want to return to the place she lost her mother. Couldn't do it. Wouldn't do it.

In 2025, that changed. My mum turned sixty in March, and we organised a big party for her at our favourite spot, Uluwatu Surf Villas. We gathered the family and thirty of Mum's friends and celebrated all that is Alyson Chapman.

The trip was a big deal for Mum, who had been so hesitant to return to Bali. I know it was healing for her, and it was healing for me too. In the mornings, before the hustle and bustle of the day, Paul would take Bobbi out to sit on the grass and look out at the ocean. My dad would go down to the beach for a surf, my mum would sleep in, and I would join Paul with a coffee. I hoped my grandma and poppa could see us. I hoped they were proud. I finally had the baby I had asked her to send me from above. Bobbi was heaven on earth.

My mum's return to Bali marked a shift. A lot changed in 2025.

After five years, I found the little brown onesie, which I bought when I was pregnant for the first time in 2020. I remember ordering the outfit and being so excited for all that was to come. I'd marvelled at how small it was, and pictured our baby wearing it. When I lost the baby, I put it away.

In the time since, I lost another three pregnancies; five babies passed without ever wearing that onesie. It sat, unworn, in the cupboard. Part of me worried the onesie would never be worn. But another part knew intuitively that it would.

When my friend Tiana gave birth to a baby boy in early 2025, I gave her the onesie from my cupboard. I hadn't known what to do with it before then; Bobbi had missed her chance to wear it because we were overseas, and she grew so quickly. I couldn't throw it away, but I didn't want to keep it hidden anymore either. I was ready to let it go.

When Patty was born, I knew I wanted to pass the onesie on to Tiana. It was a freeing moment. I wasn't just letting go of an item of clothing, I was releasing some of the pain I had held onto for half a decade.

It's a well-worn saying, but time really does heal. In more ways than one.

In the throes of labour, I was certain I would never – could never – give birth again. I was one and done. In the aftermath of labour, I was certain I would never be able to poo normally again; I was worried I would never have the strength to leave the house again; I was sure I would never have sex again. With time, all of those things changed.

Now, I would absolutely have another baby if I were lucky enough to fall pregnant again. I still have embryos on ice in Australia and the States, but I don't think I'll consider going through IVF again until Bobbi is a bit older. I want to give my daughter my everything: my attention, my love, my time. I don't want to miss a single moment of her childhood waiting in IVF clinics, getting blood tests, or crying silently in the bathroom.

As much as I've always wanted more than one child, I don't want to give up precious time with the baby I do have, trying to conceive the baby I don't have. Throughout the end of my twenties and the start of my thirties, my life revolved around my hormonal cycle, needles, egg counts and scans. My emotions see-sawed from hope to despair, joy to grief. My stomach was always bruised and my heart too often broken.

It was all worth it – for Bobbi – but I'm not racing to go through it again. Even with the distance of time.

There's a sculpture that sits on my bedside table. It's a statue of my pregnant body. Libby from SETT + MAXE came and took a 3D photo of me when I was in hospital on bed rest. I had to stand completely still – and butt naked – while she scanned every inch of my body. SETT + MAXE turned the image into a mould, and turned that mould into a work of art. It's one of the most precious things I own. When I look at the figure of my body carrying baby Bobbi, I see beauty and strength. I genuinely miss my pregnant body and the feeling of my belly.

When I look back on Bobbi's birth today, I remember how incredible it was. I remember the intense connection I had with Paul and the ridiculous amount of love I felt for him. I would go back and relive that moment over and over again if I could.

Yes, I remember the pain and the fear and the blood too, but those memories have dulled, while the others have grown brighter. And every day, I make new memories with my daughter.

When Bobbi wakes up of a morning, I go into her room to scoop her up. And every morning, she looks at me with the brightest eyes and the biggest smile. I swear she smiles so much, her face creases and her eyes close. She looks at me like I'm the sun and the moon, which makes sense, because that's how I look at her.

I love breastfeeding, which I know is incredibly fortunate. When Bobbi's on the boob, she holds my finger on one hand, and she makes me hold her foot with my other hand. Those moments of connection with her are the highlight of my day. I don't take them for granted, because I know not everyone gets to experience them. Not all mothers are able to breastfeed, and some decide not to. There is absolutely no shame in that.

If there was one thing I could change about motherhood, it's all the judgement and pressure and societal expectations. Being a mum is hard enough without side eyes and snarky comments.

This is the reality: motherhood is extreme. The highest of highs and the lowest of lows.

In the early days postpartum, I lost myself completely. I feel like I'm slowly finding myself again, but I'm not the person I once was. For better and worse. I can no longer drop everything and join Paul on the road. I can no longer work 24/7. I can no longer have a couple of glasses of wine without worrying if I'll be nursing a hangover – and a baby – in the morning. I'm more than happy to pay this price, but it's a price nonetheless. Motherhood changes everything. In my eyes, you don't have to be perfect, you just have to be present.

There's such an emphasis on 'the juggle' for mums. I don't know if it's possible to perfectly balance motherhood and work (and all the other things). So instead of focusing on keeping all my balls in the air, I'm trying to focus on my time with each ball. That was a juggling reference, but it sounds slightly dirty, I know. Regardless, the sentiment stands. When I'm with Bobbi, I try to be completely present as her mum. When I'm doing work, I try to be present in that role as well. I've found separating the two helps me show up better. If I do everything at once, I spread myself too thin.

I've started telling myself that it's okay to work, and it's okay to enjoy work. I've never not worked (remember my neighbourhood gardening club?), and I get a real sense of achievement and independence from the work that I do. 'Mum guilt' is an easy trap to fall into, but I refuse to feel guilt for providing for my family, being passionate about my job, and asking for help when I need it. We're in such a privileged position to have amazing friends and family who love Bobbi and jump at the chance to look after her. I know not everyone has that kind of support, and I'm the first to admit we wouldn't be able to live the life that we live without our community.

On an ordinary afternoon in 2025, when Bobbi was ten months old, Paul and I were hanging out with Kane, his wife, Tash, and their kids. Kane had made his famous stew, the one I'd devoured in hospital after giving birth to Bobbi, and which I'd been dreaming about ever since. Before dinner, we wandered down to Palm Beach to watch the sunset. There wasn't a lick of wind, the beach was still and the air was crisp. The sky was awash with pastels: pale blue, dusty pink, soft lavender and a warm peach. We stood with our feet in the sand as the sun slipped below the horizon. The kids played in the shallows and Bobbi smiled her sweet, sweet smile.

Three years earlier, almost to the day, Paul and I were on the same stretch of sand at Palm Beach. We weren't standing though, we were kneeling – mourning the loss of our identical twin boys with two long-stemmed, white roses. At the time, the grief floored me. I didn't know if I would ever recover from the blow.

But there I was, three years later. Standing. And smiling at my baby girl.

Bobbi has healed my deepest wounds and softened the hardened parts of me. She is the reason I believe in miracles. She is everything I dreamed of, envisioned, and begged for.

For years, I looked for reasons to keep hope. I searched for signs from the universe, I asked to be sent feathers, I spoke to my grandma, my babies and Chumpy in the sky.

The signs gave me strength and showed me a path forward. That path led straight to our baby girl.

It was always Bobbi.

EPILOGUE

THE SHOCK *ALMOST* BROUGHT ME TO MY KNEES. IT WAS TWO days before Bobbi's first birthday, and we were getting her ready for bed. We were at home in Ibiza; Paul had started his summer season at UNVRS, and I had finished the edit of this book, which was being typeset and ready for printing. Paul was rocking Bobbi to sleep in her room, and I was in the bathroom. I had been super emotional thinking about our baby's upcoming birthday. For so long, I had looked at Bobbi in amazement; I couldn't believe that she was real, and that she was ours. Then I couldn't believe that she was turning one!

Time was going too fast. I tried to rewind it by watching videos of Bobbi from when she was a newborn. I unexpectedly burst into sobs watching a video of her feeding. I had weaned Bobbi six weeks earlier. It happened naturally. We started giving Bobbi a bottle at bedtime; my milk supply decreased, and so too did the frequency of my feeds. It was an easy transition for Bobbi because she loves a bottle and didn't beg for the boob. It was much harder on me. I didn't realise how much I would miss breastfeeding. I felt a real sense of loss. My hormones were all over the place, and my tears were dangerously close to the surface. It was normal – your hormones fluctuate as your body adjusts to the end of milk production – I knew that. But understanding why I was teary didn't make me any less teary.

When I got my period back after stopping breastfeeding, it really felt like the end of a chapter. I desperately wanted to flick the pages back and stay in the moment. I had everything I ever wanted: a healthy baby, and that baby was growing up too damn quickly! Bobbi was turning into such a big girl, and I wasn't ready for it. I missed nursing her to sleep; I missed the feeling of her holding onto my finger as I fed her; I missed seeing her looking up at me while she was on the boob, staring at me like I was her whole world. Her sun and her moon.

I was thinking about all of those things that night, at bedtime, in Ibiza, in the bathroom. Suddenly it dawned on me that I hadn't had another period since it had come back, more than a month ago. I was late.

I opened the bathroom cabinet and reached for the bulk pack of pregnancy tests from summers gone by when I had prayed and prayed to see two lines. In the five years I spent trying to conceive, I can't begin to guess how many sticks I peed on, but I'll never forget how hard I squinted trying to see a second line. I used to take the sticks outside into the natural light, put my phone torch on them, take photos of them and zoom in – anxiously trying to see that precious second line.

I didn't need to squint that night, at bedtime, in Ibiza, in the bathroom. As soon as I peed on the stick, I saw two lines. They were thick and bright. My knees nearly buckled underneath me in complete shock. I had to steady myself on the sink. Somehow, I stayed upright. My eyes remained glued on the stick in front of me. I had never seen two more convincing lines; and yet, I wasn't convinced. I was sure it was a mistake, a false positive, an out-of-date test.

I immediately grabbed another test, and it immediately showed another two lines.

'Paul. . .' I called out.

He came into the bathroom holding a sleepy Bobbi in his arms. I looked at him, and looked at her, and shook my head in disbelief. 'I'm pregnant,' I said.

'How good!' he replied.

It was true. I bought a fresh pregnancy test at the pharmacy the next day, and the result was the same as the others: I was pregnant. I did the math and worked out I must have fallen pregnant in Malta – naturally – at the end of May. First the Maldives, now Malta. We clearly have a thing for countries starting with M.

When I was writing the last chapter of this book – just a few pages ago! – I said, 'As much as I've always wanted more than one child, I don't want to give up precious time with the baby I have, trying to conceive the baby I don't have.' I meant it. I wasn't in a rush to have another baby, and I wasn't ready to get back on the fertility roller-coaster. I didn't know if I could handle more rounds of IVF, further surgeries, or another loss.

In the same breath as I said all of that, I also said: 'I would absolutely have another baby if I were lucky enough to fall pregnant again.' My motto has always been, if it happens, it happens. And it happened. Again. After five years of trying every treatment, every procedure, every medication and every old-wives'-tale trick, I ended up falling pregnant naturally. Again.

Any wonder I was feeling so emotional about Bobbi's birthday. It wasn't just the weaning hormones!

I am writing this sentence on Bobbi's first birthday. My best friends and Bobbi's godmummys, Laura and Ellidy, have arrived in Ibiza just in time for the milestone. They came to celebrate one baby, and I surprised them with another . . . When the girls touched down in Ibiza – after completing The Big 5 half-marathon in the African jungle – Jaynee and I met them at UNVRS before Paul's set. I organised a bottle of champagne for us in the green room and cleared the room, so it was just the four of us girls. Jaynee already knew my secret. Laura was still doing her make-up and rubbing foundation into her face when I pulled her, Jaynee and Ell in to do a toast. It was after midnight, and officially Bobbi's birthday. 'We have so much to celebrate,' I said. 'Congratulations to you guys for doing a marathon! Congrats to Bobbi for turning one today! And another congrats to Bobbi, who will be a big sister in eight months' time!'

There was a moment of shocked silence. Then the noise hit. 'I knew it!' Ell squealed.

'Shut up, you did not,' I replied, laughing.

Laura and Ell were thrilled, and the three girls happily polished off the bottle of champagne for me.

The timing was uncanny. I had planned for a 'Hot Girl Summer.' I had survived my first year of motherhood, and I was ready to have some fun, to catch Paul's shows and to party with Laura and Ell for the few days they were in town. For a split-second, I thought, 'The baby couldn't have waited one more month!?' Then I remembered an actual sentence I had written earlier in this book: 'Babies don't give a shit about your schedule.' My plans didn't matter to the universe. It had a plan of its own. Once more, I surrendered to the powers above. I trusted that whatever was meant for me, would come to me. I saw a different future ahead. It was bright – just like the lines on the pregnancy test.

I was sure the baby inside me must have seen all the fun Bobbi was having and couldn't wait to join the party. I didn't blame them. Our life was an epic party.

Under all the giddy excitement, the nerves are ever-present. I messaged Dr Kee Ong straight away and asked him to send me the protocol I was on when I was pregnant with Bobbi. I booked in to meet with a doctor in Ibiza and do an early scan. I was only six weeks, so we couldn't see a heartbeat yet, but the doctor said the baby was in the right spot and that it wasn't ectopic. I breathed a small sigh of relief, but I didn't fully exhale. Instead, I started taking prednisone, Clexane shots, progesterone, aspirin and a prenatal supplement again. The protocol worked with Bobbi, and I hoped it would work again.

A couple of weeks later in Paris, I had some brown spotting in my underwear. It felt like I had almost been waiting for it. Every time I went to the bathroom, I checked for blood. I couldn't help it. I was too accustomed to loss. As soon as I saw the spotting, I googled: 'Brown spotting early pregnancy.' I've done a thousand different variations of that search over the years. Google told me what I already knew: brown spotting is normal in early pregnancy. I tried not to worry because the blood wasn't fresh and red; I tried to remind myself that my future was already planned; and I tried to tell myself that I would be okay if I went through another loss. My self-talk was silenced by an even louder inner voice. 'I really want this,' the voice said.

I had this naïve thought once I had Bobbi, it wouldn't matter if I didn't have another baby. Then I fell pregnant. Now I'm hoping and praying and begging the universe again, 'Please let this baby be okay.'

When I told Paul about the spotting in Paris, he gave me a look that said, 'Oh no, not again.' I don't think our fear will ever go away. I wonder if people who haven't gone through a pregnancy loss experience this same anxiety – I'll never know personally. I'm sure everyone has a level of worry, and that is amplified and elevated after a loss.

At the time of writing this, I am pregnant. I don't know if that will still be the case when the book is printed, or by the time it hits the shelves. I know – all too well – how quickly the joy of a positive pregnancy test can turn to despair. I've been here before. I don't want to get ahead of myself, or to jinx things, or to set myself up for sorrow.

I feel it all: shock, elation, fear and gratitude. Most of all, I feel hope. I am hopeful that this book will end on a happy note. I am hopeful that I'll be able to give Bobbi a little brother or sister. I am hopeful that dreams can come true twice.

When I sat down to write *Always You*, I thought Bobbi was our happy ending. But, maybe, she was only the beginning . . .

ACKNOWLEDGEMENTS

On a quiet autumn morning, I woke up before dawn to shoot the cover for this book. It was 5 am when I arrived at the beach with my friend and photographer Karina Enever, who shot Bobbi's birth and our first family photos. When I got out of the car, I stepped straight onto a long, black feather. It was fitting. Throughout my fertility journey, I looked for feathers as signs to keep going. Throughout the process of writing this book – largely about my fertility journey – I reflected on all the feathers that appeared when I needed them the most. And as I went to capture this cover image, there it was: a feather. I asked Karina to take a photo of it.

I need to start by thanking the universe for sending me so many signs and symbols of hope. Because of them, I was able to keep hold of my belief that I would be a mother. That I would have a baby. That my daughter was waiting for me.

To Paul,

My best friend, my rock, my forever. Thank you for standing by me through every heartbreak, every needle, hospital visits, and highs. You held me through it all, even when I was falling apart. Your strength gave me mine. Watching you become Bobbi's dad has been the greatest gift I've ever witnessed.

I am endlessly proud of the man you are, the father you are and all that you do for our little family. You give everything to us, even when you're running on empty. Thank you for working so hard, for loving so big, for keeping the music on and the mood light when I needed it most.

I'll never forget the way Bobbi looked at you the moment she was born, like she already knew you were her whole world. I see it every time she smiles at you now. You're her DJ, her hero, her big softie. And you're mine, too.

We love you so much.

To my mum,

Thank you for being the soft place I could land. For answering every call, no matter the time. For worrying, for hoping, for loving me fiercely. For teaching me what it means to show up, always.

To my dad,

Thank you for being the quiet strength in the background. You've always been steady, calm, and full of heart. Watching you become Bobbi's pop has been one of the sweetest joys, the way you look at Bobbi melts me. Thank you for teaching me what loyalty looks like and for being there through every chapter, even when it was hard to find the words.

To my siblings, Cooper, Olivia and Sophia,

You three have been my anchor, my cheerleaders, and my safe place all rolled into one. Thank you for loving me through every twist and turn, for showing up with hugs, humour, and the kind of loyalty only siblings can give.

I love you all so much. Bobbi is lucky to have the coolest, kindest, most solid crew of aunties and uncle around her.

To my grandparents, Poppa and Grandma,

Even though you're no longer here, your love still surrounds me.

Thank you for showing me the world, for shaping who I am and for teaching me what love truly looks like.

I wish you got to meet Bobbi – you would've adored her, and she would've loved you right back.

I carry you with me, always.

To Bobbi's godmummys, Ellidy and Laura,

You are two of the most important women in my life and I couldn't imagine anyone more perfect to help guide and love my girl.

Ellidy, you've been in it with me since the very beginning, through the heartbreak, the miracles, the chaos and the beauty. You were there when Bobbi was born and you've been by my side ever since. You spoil her with cuddles, cute outfits and a love so strong it makes my heart burst. But more than that, you've cared for *me*. You've held me, protected me, made me laugh when I didn't think I could. You're not just Bobbi's god mummy, you're family.

Laura, you've been my best mate since I was five and now you're my daughter's god mother, so special. You bring this spark, this sunshine, this joy that Bobbi already responds to in the most beautiful way. You always know when I need checking in on, when I need a giggle or a pep talk or a wine. You've got the rarest kind of magic, and I hope Bobbi grows up with that same wild, beautiful energy.

Thank you both for loving her and for loving me, too. For showing up. For never missing a beat. Bobbi is so lucky to have you both and I'm so lucky to have you as my sisters in life.

To Minnie,

Our girl. Our first baby. You might not have come from my belly, but you live in my heart like you always have. You made me a mum in so many ways, long before Bobbi arrived.

Watching you meet your baby sister was one of the most special moments of my life. You came bursting into that hospital room with flowers in your hands and sparkles in your eyes and you've been loving 'your baby Bobbi' ever since.

Thank you for being the best big sister, for the cuddles, the giggles, the 'gentle' pats on her head, and for calling her 'your baby'. Thank you for being patient with us as we learned to juggle life with a newborn. And thank you for loving Paul and me with your whole heart.

Your 'Bobbi boots' will always remind me of the way you lit up that day. I hope you always know how important you are to our little family. We love you more than words can ever say.

To Karina,

Thank you for capturing some of the most sacred moments of my life, my pregnancy, Bobbi's birth and the cover of this very book. Your lens has held my story with such softness, strength and intention.

You've witnessed me at my most vulnerable and my most empowered and somehow, you've managed to bottle all of that emotion into your work. You've been more than a photographer, you've been a calming presence, a creative force and a true friend throughout this journey.

I'm so grateful for your magic, your eye and your heart. These images will stay with me forever.

To Bobbi's goddaddy, Kane,

Thank you for loving our girl like your own and for showing up for me in such a big way.

From cooking me meals in those hazy early postpartum days to keeping the mood light and fun when I needed it most, you were exactly what we needed. Your energy, your heart, and your hilarious sense of humour brought so much joy into our little newborn bubble. Bobbi absolutely adores you (and so do we).

To Brett,

You've been more than just Paul's manager, you've been one of our rocks. Thank you for holding it down for us during the wildest seasons, for protecting Paul when he needed space to be present and for always having our family's back. You've shown up in big ways and quiet ones and we've never taken that for granted.

In a world that moves fast and never slows down, your loyalty, honesty, and care have meant everything. We trust you with the business, but more than that, we trust you with *us*.

To Tallara,

We love you and we're so lucky to have you in our corner. Thank you for caring for me through some of my hardest moments. You looked after me post my biggest surgery in the US with so much love, patience and gentleness. I'll never forget how safe and supported you made me feel when I needed it most. Forever grateful for you.

To Jenn,

You're our backbone, our sounding board, and our confidante. Thank you for keeping everything (and everyone!) running smoothly, for believing in us, and for always being the calm in the chaos. We're so lucky to have you in our corner.

To Bella,

You stepped in late in the piece, but you've supported me like you've been here from the very beginning. You've worked tirelessly to bring this dream to life and you've done it with so much care, clarity, and commitment. Thank you for holding space for me through it all.

To Jaynee and Richie,

Richie, you've been part of this story from the very beginning. You believed in me before this book was even a thing, and you helped bring it to life – literally. Your support has never wavered, and I'm so thankful for you. Jaynee, my soul sister – thank you for being one of my biggest supporters and best friends. You've shown up in all the ways that matter – in real life, in real moments, and always just one call away. Your love, honesty, and loyalty mean everything to me.

To the midwives and nurses at John Flynn Hospital, especially Lisa, Clare and Gaylene, and to every doctor and embryologist who played a part in our journey,

Thank you for your work, your care, your compassion. Especially to Clare and Lisa – you both quite literally saved my life.

To Dr Kee Ong, my fertility specialist, and Dr Camran Nezhat, my surgeon,

Thank you for your care, your expertise, and your belief in me. You both played such an important role in my journey to motherhood, and I will be forever grateful.

Dr Trueman, my obstetrician,

Thank you for your guidance, your calm presence, and for safely delivering our precious Bobbi. Your care throughout my pregnancy and birth gave me so much reassurance, even in the scariest moments. I'll be forever grateful to you for helping bring her into the world.

To K, our surrogate,

Thank you for the selfless love and courage you showed in being willing to carry our baby. Even though the journey didn't unfold the way we expected, your heart, your support, and your belief in our dream meant everything to us.

You were a light in one of our darkest seasons and I'll always be grateful for the role you played in our story.

My *Darling, Shine!* family and everyone who shared their own stories with me along the way,

Thank you for being the heartbeat of this journey.

To our listeners, our community and every single person who's messaged, hugged, cried with or opened up to me. Your stories, your bravery, and your vulnerability have meant more than I can say. You reminded me that I'm not alone, even in the darkest moments.

You all helped me find the strength to keep going and the courage to share my own story out loud. This book belongs to every woman who's ever whispered, *me too.*

To Daisy (@spiritualmixtape) and Faye (@manowai.rituals),

Thank you for holding such beautiful space for me at my baby showers as I stepped into motherhood. Daisy, your blessing in LA was pure magic. Faye, your circle in Australia grounded me deeply. I'll carry the energy of those moments with me forever.

To my Hachette team, Vanessa Radnidge, Lee Moir, Vanessa Lanaway, Bethany Neville, Emily Lighezzolo and the incredible crew behind the scenes,

Thank you for helping me bring this book to life with integrity and heart. You've honoured my story with care and creativity and I'm so grateful.

To Alley,

This book simply wouldn't exist without you.

Thank you for helping me find the words when I didn't know where to start and for honouring my story with so much care, patience and heart. You've taken the most personal, emotional, and vulnerable chapters of my life and helped me shape them into something that feels true, powerful, and *me*.

You've written so many pieces on me over the years, but this one means the most. Thank you for listening so deeply, holding space so gently, and bringing this story to life in the most beautiful way.

I'm so grateful for you! Your talent, your calm, and your belief in me. What a gift you've given.

To the babies I never got to hold,

You changed me. You opened my heart to motherhood in a way I never saw coming. You are written into every page.

This book is for the ones still hoping, still waiting, still grieving,

You are not alone.

You are not broken.

You are so deeply loved.

And lastly, to my daughter, Bobbi Maree,

You are the light that made all the darkness worth it. My rainbow. My magic. My everything.

This book exists because of you – and for you. It was *Always You.*

I hope one day, when you're old enough to understand, you'll read these pages and feel just how deeply you were wished for, fought for and loved.

You were the dream I never let go of. And the moment I held you, I knew, every single step led me to you. You made me a mother. You made me whole.

If you are holding this book and made it this far, *thank you.*

With all my heart,

Chloe Maree Fisher

Xxx

RESOURCES

No-one should have to walk the journey of miscarriage and pregnancy alone – there is help and support available.

PINK ELEPHANTS

The Pink Elephants support network provides help, guidance and information for those who've experienced early pregnancy loss. The organisation offers a peer support live chat, a pregnancy loss helpline, a bereavement support program and various Circle communities, where you can connect with others who have experienced a similar loss. You can read about how Pink Elephants started in the Appendix. Founder Samantha Payne has generously shared her story.

www.pinkelephants.org.au

FERTILITY SOCIETY AUSTRALIA AND NEW ZEALAND

The Fertility Society of Australia and New Zealand (FSANZ) is the peak body representing scientists, doctors, researchers, nurses, counsellors and patients in reproductive medicine in Australia and New Zealand. Their objective is to provide clinical guidance to improve the standard of reproductive medical practice, and as such, they have a wealth of knowledge in the space. For anyone considering fertility treatment and wanting to know about the process, the information shared by FSANZ is a solid place to start.

www.fertilitysociety.com.au

PANDA

Perinatal Anxiety and Depression Australia (PANDA) operates Australia's only National Perinatal Mental Health Helpline for individuals, their families, support people and health care providers. Their phone and online services provide access to counselling and information to support the mental health and wellbeing of people who are planning, starting or raising a family.

www.panda.org.au
PANDA National Helpline (Monday to Saturday) 1300 726 306

GIDGET FOUNDATION

The Gidget Foundation is a not-for-profit organisation that raises awareness of Perinatal Anxiety and Depression and supports the emotional wellbeing of expectant, new and potential parents.

They offer face-to-face services at their Gidget House centres in New South Wales, Queensland, Tasmania, Victoria and Western Australia, as well as telehealth counselling services nationally.

www.gidgetfoundation.org.au
1300 851 758

COPE – CENTRE OF PERINATAL EXCELLENCE

The eCOPE Directory – put together by COPE – is a national database of services that provide perinatal expertise. You can search for health professionals in your area and see information on waitlist times, types of services and cost structure.

www.cope.org.au/e-cope-directory

DARLING, SHINE! COMMUNITY

The *Darling, Shine!* Facebook group is a community of likeminded women who offer each other support, guidance and (asked for) advice on everything from fertility, grief, miscarriage and pregnancy, to fashion, baby products, gift ideas and Bali recommendations. We have a dedicated IVF Support group chat, and a chat for giving and getting support.

www.facebook.com/groups/darlingshinecommunity

Appendix

THE BEGINNING OF PINK ELEPHANTS

Pink Elephants Support Network CEO Samantha Payne has generously shared her story, and I'm so pleased to be able to include it here.

'I'm sorry, there is no heartbeat.'

The sentence that changed my life.

2015 – nine years

2016 – eight years

2020 – four years

These are the ages of the children I don't get the privilege of parenting; their due and death dates forever etched on my heart. Loved and wanted babies, who didn't survive pregnancy.

In between those dates, there are the dates of the three babies I did manage to welcome safely in my arms. I'm acutely aware of how privileged I am to have my children Georgie, Johnny and Rose. But the arrival of one baby doesn't take away the loss of another. The loss always remains. I spent a decade trying to build my family, falling pregnant and losing loved babies.

I am still traumatised by the lack of empathy and care I was shown at times, and the neglect that led to traumatic experiences like deciding to flush the remains of my ten-week baby down the toilet as I miscarried 'naturally' at home. Or the number of times I was told 'at least it was early' or 'it's nature's way, there was probably something wrong with it'. These commonly said sentences only served to compound my grief and isolate me from seeking support. I felt so ashamed after my second miscarriage. *Why can't I do something that is meant to be so natural? Why do my babies keep dying? Am I such an awful mother to my firstborn that I don't deserve to have another baby?*

When I left hospital after my first – and second and third – miscarriages, I went home empty. I was not given a guide on what to expect or how to navigate my grief. I was on my own and entirely lost.

I wanted to honour those babies, and to create change for Georgie, Johnny and Rose. I carry on the work I do because I'll be damned if they go through miscarriage in the future in the way that I did.

Pink Elephants, a support network and advocacy collective, is now nearly a decade old, and we've achieved some incredible milestones that I will forever be proud of. We have championed and changed federal legislation in Australia, resulting in the *Fair Work Act 2009* being amended to include miscarriage under bereavement leave. We've directly supported hundreds of thousands of women like me who deserve a circle of support, to offer them validation, empathy and connection when they are in the depths of grief after losing their loved babies or anxiety-inducing subsequent pregnancies. This year, we've also received $4 million in funding from the Department of Health and Aged Care to scale and expand support for miscarriage services and mental health care. It is our first government funding – we've had to rely entirely on donations – and it's going to make such an enormous difference.

People now talk about their experiences of miscarriage more openly. When Chloe started to publicly speak about pregnancy loss in 2020, I immediately connected with her story. She spoke from a place of vulnerability and made space for other women to speak from that place too. There's strength in that. I invited Chloe to sit on the board of Pink Elephants so we can keep facilitating these important conversations about infertility and miscarriage.

For those currently going through loss, please know, it's not your fault. You didn't do anything wrong. You are allowed to grieve the loss of your baby. You can ask for support; Pink Elephants exists for you.

Knowing how much I wish I'd had these resources to help me, I am very proud to be part of the Pink Elephants board and have such respect for the work Samantha is doing. Remember, there are resources and people to support you.

PICTURE SECTION CAPTIONS

PICTURE SECTION ONE

Page 1

Top row and middle left: Me with my mum, and with Poppa and Grandma just after I was born.
Middle right: Lots of people think Bobbi looks like a mini me. I can see a little of both me and Paul. But she is more and more her own person.
Bottom row: My first day at kindy.

Page 2

The beach was where it was at for my family, and we spent a lot of time swimming, surfing and at nippers – at least until the great seaweed incident put me off surfing! But never off the beach.

Page 3

Top left: Grandma and me.
Top right: Dad, Olivia, Sophia and me.
Middle: Cooper, Sophia, me, Grandma and Olivia.
Bottom left: Laura and I starting early!
Bottom middle: My bestie, my ride or die, the magnificent Laura Enever. We were forever putting on a show.

Pages 4 and 5

My friends and family make my world go round. Good or bad, we're always there for each other.

Pages 6 and 7

From the moment we met, he was the one.

Page 8

Middle left: I'll always cherish this photo of my grandma with the roses at my wedding.

Middle right: Honouring her and trying to deal with our grief.

Bottom left: Our little flat on Narrabeen Lake.

Bottom right: My family, my loves – Dad, Olivia, Sophia, me, Mum and Cooper.

PICTURE SECTION TWO

Pages 1 and 2

I like nothing more than spreadsheets and organising, which comes in very handy when you start a business. From Aloe Swimwear to Hard Fizz and *Darling, Shine!*, I've loved every second of it.

Page 3

On the road touring with Paul.

Middle left: I had to include this Grammys shot! And I still think Paul was robbed.

Pages 4 and 5

My IVF and pregnancy journey. The highest of highs, and the lowest of lows.

Page 6

Welcome to the world, Bobbi Maree!

Page 7

Ellidy and I love that Bobbi and Minnie are going to grow up together.

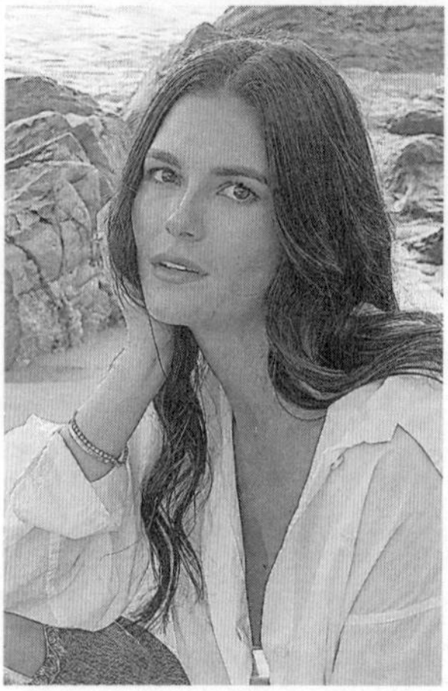

Chloe Fisher is a businesswoman, entrepreneur and podcaster. She juggles her career and motherhood alongside being the number one tour partner for her husband FISHER, the Grammy-nominated international DJ. Her multiple ventures include Australian Seltzer brand Hard Fizz and the *Darling, Shine!* podcast. Chloe is also on the board of the Pink Elephants Support Network, a not-for-profit that provides resources, information and peer-support for anyone impacted by early pregnancy loss. She uses her powerful voice and social platforms to provide a voice for women struggling with infertility. Chloe splits her time between the Gold Coast, Ibiza, LA and Europe. *Always You* is her first book.

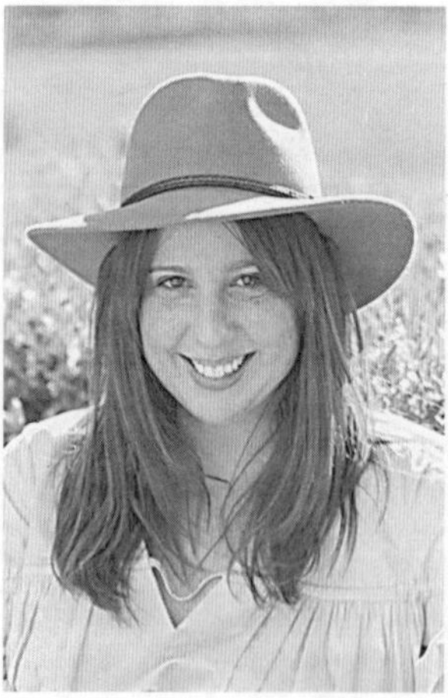

Alley Pascoe is a bestselling, award-winning writer with a background in magazines and memoirs. Her books include the acclaimed *Heartstrong* with Ellidy Pullin, *Love and Pain* with Ben Gillies and Chris Joannou of Silverchair, *The Girl in the Green Dress* with Jeni Haynes and *There Must Be More* with Kellie Finlayson.